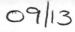
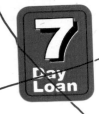

DEVELOPING

ENDURANCE

National Strength and Conditioning Association

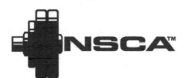

Ben Reuter

EDITOR

Human Kinetics

Library of Congress Cataloging-in-Publication Data

Developing endurance / National Strength and Conditioning Association (NSCA) ; Ben Reuter, editor.
   p. cm. -- (Sport performance series)
 Includes bibliographical references and index.
 ISBN-13: 978-0-7360-8327-0 (soft cover)
 ISBN-10: 0-7360-8327-8 (soft cover)
 1. Physical fitness. 2. Physical education and training--Physiological aspects. 3. Exercise--Physiological aspects. 4. Endurance sports. I. Reuter, Ben. II. National Strength & Conditioning Association (U.S.)
 GV481.D47 2012
 613.7--dc23

                   2011044117

ISBN-10: 0-7360-8327-8 (print)
ISBN-13: 978-0-7360-8327-0 (print)

Developmental Editor: Heather Healy; **Assistant Editor:** Claire Marty; **Copyeditor:** Pat Connolly; **Indexer:** Nan N. Badgett; **Permissions Manager:** Martha Gullo; **Graphic Designer:** Joe Buck; **Cover Designer:** Keith Blomberg; **Photographer (cover):** ©Human Kinetics; **Photographer (interior):** Neil Bernstein, ©Human Kinetics, unless otherwise noted; **Photo Asset Manager:** Laura Fitch; **Visual Production Assistant:** Joyce Brumfield; **Photo Production Manager:** Jason Allen; **Art Manager:** Kelly Hendren; **Associate Art Manager:** Alan L. Wilborn; **Illustrations:** © Human Kinetics, unless otherwise noted; **Printer:** United Graphics

We thank the National Strength and Conditioning Association in Colorado Springs, Colorado, for assistance in providing the location for the photo shoot for this book.

Human Kinetics books are available at special discounts for bulk purchase. Special editions or book excerpts can also be created to specification. For details, contact the Special Sales Manager at Human Kinetics.

Printed in the United States of America   10 9 8 7 6 5 4 3 2 1

The paper in this book is certified under a sustainable forestry program.

Human Kinetics
Website: www.HumanKinetics.com

United States: Human Kinetics
P.O. Box 5076
Champaign, IL 61825-5076
800-747-4457
e-mail: humank@hkusa.com

Canada: Human Kinetics
475 Devonshire Road Unit 100
Windsor, ON N8Y 2L5
800-465-7301 (in Canada only)
e-mail: info@hkcanada.com

Europe: Human Kinetics
107 Bradford Road
Stanningley
Leeds LS28 6AT, United Kingdom
+44 (0) 113 255 5665
e-mail: hk@hkeurope.com

Australia: Human Kinetics
57A Price Avenue
Lower Mitcham, South Australia 5062
08 8372 0999
e-mail: info@hkaustralia.com

New Zealand: Human Kinetics
P.O. Box 80
Torrens Park, South Australia 5062
0800 222 062
e-mail: info@hknewzealand.com

E4819

DEVELOPING ENDURANCE

Contents

Introduction

Participation in endurance sports and racing is a growing activity for people all over the world. In many countries, a popular recreational activity is participating in running races and triathlons to raise money for charitable organizations. More and more people are participating in 10K runs, marathons, and bike tours. A growing number of people are also participating in triathlon races ranging from sprint distances to Ironman. Additionally, noncompetitive bike tours, triathlons, marathons, adventure races, and other types of prolonged aerobic activity attract people from diverse backgrounds.

Knowledge of proper training programs and techniques for endurance training is still catching up with participation. A training program that is properly designed is essential for athletes to be able to enjoy endurance activities as much as possible. A properly designed program can also minimize the risk of injury and maximize performance for those individuals who are competing.

Many endurance activities involve some amount of running. According to various research studies, as many as 75 to 80 percent of runners are injured each year; an injury is defined as something that causes the runner to miss one or more days of training. Often these injuries occur because of improperly designed training and conditioning programs. The information provided in this book can be a valuable tool to help the endurance coach or self-coached athlete develop a training program that is designed to maximize performance and minimize the risk of injury.

When training for endurance events, many people do not consider the importance of overall physical fitness. Physical fitness consists of three main training components: cardiovascular (or aerobic) training, resistance training, and flexibility training. Each component has a valuable place in a properly designed program for the endurance athlete.

Endurance sports are activities that require a high level of muscle endurance. This is achieved primarily through aerobic activities—running, cycling, swimming, and so on. The muscles are trained to contract repeatedly at a submaximal level without fatiguing. Some endurance training programs focus almost exclusively on aerobic training, using a "more is better" approach. This approach often leads to the exclusion of other aspects of fitness because athletes and coaches think they don't have time to devote to other areas.

Well-trained endurance athletes do need a high level of aerobic conditioning, but long-term avoidance or minimization of the other components of overall fitness—especially resistance training—can lead to performance plateaus and chronic injuries. Most people who participate in endurance sports are recreational athletes, so overall physical fitness is an important part of maintaining a high quality of life. As a person ages, muscle strength (the ability to produce force) and muscle power (the ability to produce force rapidly) decrease. Endurance training maximizes the ability to produce repeated submaximal muscle contractions, but it does very little to maintain or increase muscle strength or power.

Endurance sports are a unique activity. Participants in endurance sports have a wide range of body types, age, and experience. For example, it isn't unusual for marathoners to finish in times ranging from less than 2 1/2 hours to almost 7 hours. The age of these finishers often ranges from less than 20 years old to well over 70 years of age. Some of the participants are first-time finishers, but other participants may have previously completed numerous marathon races. No matter what the body type, age, or experience, all the athletes complete the same event over the same terrain. Each participant needs to have adequate physical conditioning, skill, and mental fortitude to ensure that he or she is able to successfully complete the event. The information in this book will benefit everyone from the novice who trains for health and fitness to the experienced competitor who is trying to maximize performance.

This book is designed for the self-coached athlete, the personal trainer interested in increasing the number of clients, and the endurance coach who is looking to review or expand knowledge. The individuals using this book may be looking to improve their competition performance, or they may be involved in endurance activities simply for enjoyment, with no intention of ever competing in an official event or competition.

Traditionally, endurance coaches and athletes may not have been aware of the National Strength and Conditioning Association (NSCA) or may not have known that NSCA members could offer training knowledge relevant to endurance athletes. By the same token, many NSCA members may not have recognized that their knowledge and skills would be valuable to endurance athletes. However, this book takes advantage of each contributor's expertise. All of the contributors were selected not only for their professional knowledge but also because they practice what they preach. The About the Contributors section at the end of the book shows that the contributors are not only experts on endurance training programs but also active participants in endurance sports.

Chapter 1 provides an overview of physiology as it pertains to physical activity. It also provides information related specifically to endurance activity, which will be especially valuable for those readers without a background in endurance sports. Chapter 2 covers testing and assessment and provides a valuable source of information that athletes, coaches, and fitness professionals can use to determine if a program is optimally effective.

Chapter 3 provides a summary of endurance training principles with an emphasis on explaining proper program design through periodization, or the systematic manipulation of exercise parameters (volume, intensity, and duration). Periodized training is designed to maximize healthy physiological adaptations and minimize the negative effects of too much exercise or too little recovery. Chapter 4 includes important information about nutrition and hydration.

Chapters 5 is an excellent introduction to training program design specific to endurance sports, including running, cycling, swimming, and triathlon. This chapter is a valuable tool for the experienced and inexperienced endurance athlete or coach. Unlike many books about endurance training, which have minimal information on resistance training, this book contains details on how resistance training can enhance the endurance athlete's training and performance. Chapter 6 provides explanations of resistance training exercises, and chapter 7 explores the science behind resistance training for the endurance athlete. These two chapters provide a clear rationale for the inclusion of resistance training in an endurance program, as well as practical direction about how to integrate the resistance training with the aerobic training.

Chapters 8 through 11 address running, cycling, swimming, and triathlon individually. These chapters include sample training programs and extensive information on sport-specific program design.

Endurance sports are a growing activity worldwide, and the dissemination of knowledge to coaches and participants of those sports is essential to make the sports as safe and enjoyable as possible. This book is an excellent addition to the library of endurance athletes, participants, and coaches who recognize the importance of training information supported by science.

CHAPTER 1

Physiology of Endurance Sport Training

Randy Wilber

This chapter provides you with the basic knowledge of exercise physiology needed for coaching or participating in endurance-based sporting activities. Understanding this information is important for people who are active competitors or people who participate in endurance activities for health and recreation. A significant amount of physical energy is required when a person trains for and competes in endurance-based sporting events. Therefore, we begin this chapter with a discussion of energy production. Some basic questions will get us started:

▶ What exactly is energy?

▶ How is energy produced and used in an endurance athlete's body?

The answers to these questions rely primarily on the basic sciences of biology and biochemistry. If you're studying these subjects for the first time, you may find them to be very technical and a bit overwhelming. In that case, you should focus on the nonscientific analogies provided and should refer to the figures where indicated. These tips will help you get the most out of this chapter.

THREE ENERGY SYSTEMS

The basic unit of energy within the human body is adenosine triphosphate (ATP). To make things simple, think of a molecule of ATP as an "energy dollar bill." Each of us has millions of molecules of ATP in our body, providing us with energy. We are constantly using and replenishing ATP, even when we are not exercising. Based on this cash analogy, ATP utilization and production can be seen as similar to the daily scenario in which we spend and earn cash to maintain our lifestyle.

The molecular structure of ATP is shown in figure 1.1. ATP is made up of three unique subunits: (1) adenine, (2) ribose, and (3) the phosphate groups. Rather than memorize the structure of ATP, focus your attention on the wavy lines that connect the three phosphate groups. Each of these wavy lines represents a high-energy bond.

Figure 1.2 shows the basic biochemical reaction whereby ATP produces energy. A single molecule of ATP is represented on the left side of the reaction. When ATP comes in contact with water and the enzyme ATPase, one of its high-energy bonds is broken or cleaved, which releases a burst of chemical energy. This burst of chemical energy can be used for all of the important physiological functions, including nerve transmission, blood circulation, tissue synthesis, glandular secretion, digestion, and skeletal muscle contraction (which we will focus on later in this chapter). When this reaction breaks the bond in ATP, it creates a molecule of adenosine diphosphate (ADP) and a phosphate molecule (P_i).

Now that you understand what energy is, let's take a look at how it is produced. The body has three energy-producing systems (see figure 1.3): the immediate (ATP-CP),

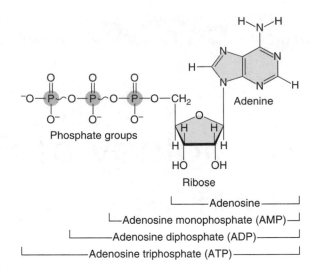

Figure 1.1 Structure of adenosine triphosphate (ATP).

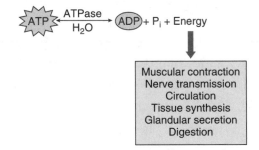

Figure 1.2 Biochemical conversion of ATP to ADP + P_i + energy.

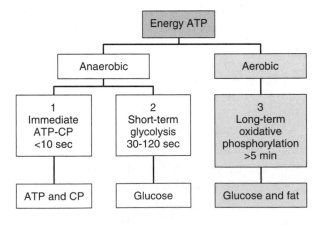

Figure 1.3 The three energy systems.

short-term (glycolysis), and long-term (oxidative phosphorylation) systems. The three energy systems are similar in that they all produce ATP, but they differ in how quickly they produce ATP and in the amount of ATP produced. Two of the three energy systems—the immediate and short-term systems—are anaerobic energy systems. In other words, these two energy systems do not require oxygen to produce ATP. In contrast, the long-term energy system is aerobic and requires oxygen to produce ATP.

The technical name for the immediate energy system is the ATP-CP system (ATP stands for adenosine triphosphate, and CP stands for creatine phosphate). The biochemical reactions involved in the immediate energy system are shown in figure 1.4. Notice that the first reaction is the same one that was described earlier for the conversion of ATP to chemical energy. Again, one of the high-energy bonds is cleaved (broken) in that reaction. As a result, ATP, which

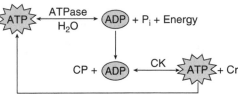

Figure 1.4 The two basic biochemical reactions of the immediate energy system (ATP-CP): (1) the synthesis of ATP from ADP and a phosphate and (2) the release of energy by the breakdown of ATP to ADP.

contains three phosphate groups, is converted to adenosine diphosphate (ADP), which contains two phosphate groups. As shown in figure 1.4, ADP is not simply thrown away after the initial reaction. Rather, it goes through a recycling process with CP (which has one phosphate group). The CP donates its phosphate group to ADP (two phosphate groups) to produce a new molecule of ATP (three phosphate groups), leaving a molecule of creatine (CR), which will later bond with another molecule of phosphate.

Using our cash analogy, the immediate energy system is similar to the cash in a person's wallet:

▶ The person can access and use the cash immediately.

▶ However, the person has a very limited amount of cash.

Similarly, the immediate energy system has the advantage of producing ATP very quickly, but it has the disadvantage of producing a very limited supply of ATP. In terms of athletic performance, the immediate energy system is the dominant energy system during very high-intensity, short-duration exercise lasting approximately 10 seconds or less. Examples of athletic events in which the immediate energy system is dominant would include the 100-meter sprint in track, a 10-meter diving event, and weightlifting events.

Like the immediate energy system, the short-term energy system is anaerobic. The technical name for the short-term energy system is glycolysis because the first of several biochemical reactions in this energy system involves the conversion of glycogen (stored glucose) to free glucose. A simplified version of the short-term energy system is shown in figure 1.5. One molecule of glucose is converted to two molecules of pyruvic acid; then, in the absence of oxygen, the two molecules of pyruvic acid are converted to two molecules of lactic acid. Most important, notice that two molecules of ATP are also produced.

Using our cash analogy, the short-term energy system is similar to the money that a person has in a checking account:

▶ The person has a larger amount of money available (compared to the cash in the person's wallet).

▶ However, accessing this money in order to transfer it into cash form takes a little longer.

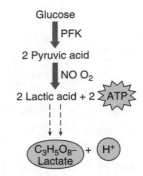

Figure 1.5 A simplified version of the biochemical reactions involving the short-term energy system (glycolysis). (PFK stands for phosphofructokinase.)

Similarly, the short-term energy system has the advantage of producing more ATP than the immediate energy system, but it has the disadvantage of taking a little more time to do so. Another disadvantage is that the short-term energy system produces lactic acid, which is quickly converted to lactate and positively charged hydrogen ions (H⁺) (refer to figure 1.5). High concentrations of H⁺ create the acidic burning sensation in exercising skeletal muscle and contribute (along with other biochemical, neural, and biomechanical factors) to premature fatigue. In terms of athletic performance, the short-term energy system is the dominant energy system during high-intensity, moderate-duration exercise lasting approximately 30 to 120 seconds. Examples include the 400-meter sprint in track, the 100-meter sprint in swimming, and the 1,000-meter track event in cycling.

The long-term energy system is aerobic in nature and requires oxygen to produce ATP. The technical name for this energy system is oxidative phosphorylation. A simplified version of this relatively complex energy system is shown in figure 1.6. Notice that the long-term energy system starts out the same way as the short-term energy system—that is, a single molecule of glucose is converted to two molecules of pyruvic acid. However, because oxygen is available, pyruvic acid is not converted to lactic acid as in the short-term energy system. Rather, pyruvic acid enters several mitochondria in the cell (see figure 1.7) and is converted to acetyl coenzyme A (acetyl CoA); it then goes through a series of biochemical reactions (Krebs cycle and electron transport system [ETS]) that ultimately produce 32 molecules of ATP.

Using our cash analogy, the long-term energy system is similar to the money that a person has placed in long-term investments such as mutual funds, stocks, bonds, or IRAs:

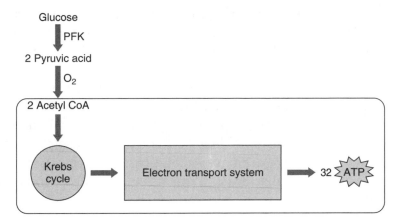

Figure 1.6 A simplified version of the biochemical reactions involved in the long-term energy system (oxidative phosphorylation). (PFK stands for phosphofructokinase.)

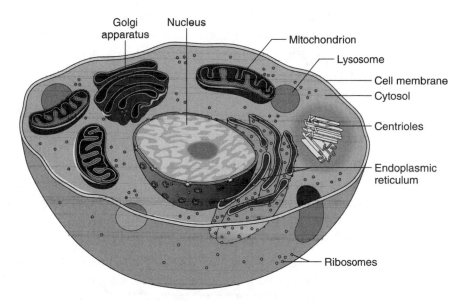

Figure 1.7 Cell structure showing several mitochondria.

▶ The person has a significantly larger amount of money compared to the money in a checking account or the cash in a wallet.

▶ However, the person must go through several more steps and must wait longer to access the funds, liquefy them, and turn them into cash.

Similarly, the long-term energy system has the advantage of producing very large amounts of ATP compared with the other energy systems; however, this system has the disadvantage of taking more time than the other energy systems to produce that large amount of ATP. The long-term energy system takes longer because it uses oxygen to produce ATP. The only place in the cell where oxygen can be used to produce ATP is in the mitochondrion, which is essentially a very large ATP factory with several "stops on the assembly line." This ultimately increases the time needed for the final production of ATP.

In terms of athletic performance, the long-term energy system is the dominant energy system in low- to moderate-intensity, long-duration exercise lasting longer than 5 minutes. Examples of this type of activity include the marathon, the 800-meter swim, and road events in cycling. So the long-term energy system is the dominant energy system used during endurance-based sporting events. However, athletes need to understand that the long-term system is not the only energy system used in endurance sports.

ENERGY DYNAMICS DURING EXERCISE

As described previously, ATP (energy) can be produced via three energy systems. Although we looked at each of the energy systems separately, this does not mean that only one energy system can function at a time. To understand this concept better, we can use the analogy of a symphony orchestra: The orchestra includes several instrument groups, and each group plays softly, moderately, or loudly depending on the musical score.

At the beginning of the symphony, the string group may be loud, the woodwind group may be moderate, and the percussion group may be soft. These musical emphases may be reversed by the end of the symphony to reflect soft music by the string group and loud music by the percussion group. The same is true for energy production during exercise. Each of the three energy systems is in a state of dynamic flux. Like the instrument groups, each of the energy systems is operating constantly during exercise, but the systems operate at different levels of ATP production depending on the intensity and duration of the exercise.

An example of the "symphony orchestra" effect is shown in figure 1.8, which shows energy dynamics during a cycling road race, a sporting event that is classified as endurance event. During pack riding, the exercise intensity is moderate, and the duration is relatively long. As discussed earlier, the dominant energy system during moderate-intensity, long-duration exercise is the long-term (oxidative phosphorylation) energy system. Although the long-term system is dominant, it is not the only energy system that is active during pack riding. The other two energy systems are active, but they are "playing softly."

During a hill climb, the intensity picks up, but the duration is shorter compared with pack riding. This type of high-intensity, moderate-duration exercise requires the short-term (glycolysis) energy system to play the loudest, the immediate (ATP-CP) energy system to play louder, and the long-term system to play softer. Finally, the energy dynamics are reversed during the final sprint to the finish, which involves exercise at a very high intensity but for a short duration. In this phase, the immediate system is clearly the loudest, and the short-term and long-term systems are relatively quiet.

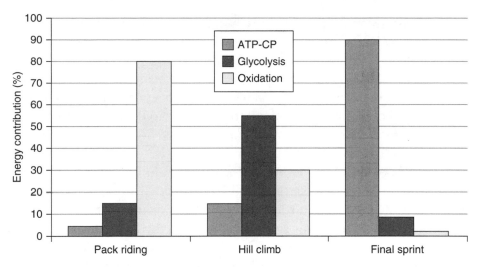

Figure 1.8 Energy dynamics during a cycling road race.

In endurance sport, the dominant energy system is the oxidative phosphorylation energy system. However, keeping in mind our symphony orchestra analogy, athletes must remember the role that the ATP-CP and glycolysis energy systems play in the performance of endurance activities. Knowing when to train and how much time to devote to training each of the three energy systems is an important ingredient of success in endurance sport. This knowledge is also reflected in a well-designed and scientifically based training plan. (Chapter 3 addresses this concept in more detail.)

CARDIOPULMONARY PHYSIOLOGY

Because endurance-based sport relies heavily on the oxidative phosphorylation energy system, endurance athletes need to understand the basic concepts of cardiopulmonary physiology. The term *cardiopulmonary* refers to the heart and lungs and how those vital organs work in synchrony to ensure that the blood is carrying oxygen and nutrients to the working skeletal muscles during exercise.

Cardiopulmonary Anatomy

The primary anatomical structures of the cardiopulmonary system are the lungs, heart, and skeletal muscles. We begin our anatomical "tour" in the lungs. Blood passes through the capillary beds of the lungs, where it unloads carbon dioxide (CO_2) and picks up oxygen (O_2). This oxygen-enriched blood travels from the lungs to the heart via the pulmonary vein. Oxygen-enriched blood initially enters the heart in the left atrium and then flows into the left ventricle. When the heart contracts, or beats, oxygen-enriched blood is ejected from the left ventricle and exits the heart via the aorta. The aorta ultimately branches into several smaller arteries that carry oxygen-enriched blood to the entire body.

Once the oxygen-enriched blood reaches, for example, the leg muscles during running, it unloads oxygen and picks up carbon dioxide. Blood exiting the exercising muscles is "oxygen reduced" and returns to the heart via the venous system. Oxygen-reduced blood is ultimately delivered to the heart via two large veins, the superior and inferior vena cava. The venae cavae deliver oxygen-reduced blood to the right atrium of the heart; the blood then flows into the right ventricle. When the heart contracts, oxygen-reduced blood is ejected by the right ventricle and travels via the pulmonary artery to the lungs.

We have now arrived back at the starting point of our tour of cardiopulmonary anatomy—that is, as the oxygen-reduced blood enters the capillary beds of the lungs, it will unload carbon dioxide and pick up oxygen and then exit the lungs as oxygen-enriched blood. This synchrony between the lungs, heart, and tissues is taking place constantly, whether the person is awake or asleep. The entire cardiopulmonary system works overtime during any endurance-based sporting activity, such as a triathlon.

Oxygen Transport

As mentioned earlier, endurance-based sports are heavily dependent on the oxidative phosphorylation energy system for ATP. In the previous section, we referred to oxygen transport in very general terms: oxygen-enriched and oxygen-reduced blood. In this section, we examine oxygen transport in more detail, focusing on the gas physics and physiology of oxygen transport.

The first thing to consider when learning about oxygen transport is how oxygen is carried around in the body. Though a very small percentage of oxygen travels through the body dissolved in the fluid portion of the blood, the primary way by which oxygen is transported through the body is via the red blood cells, also called erythrocytes. Figure 1.9 shows the shape of a typical red blood cell. Blood contains trillions of red blood cells. The portion of the blood containing red blood cells is referred to as the hematocrit (Hct) and is expressed as a percentage of volume of red blood cells relative to the total blood volume. Hematocrits for healthy individuals residing at low elevation range from 35 to 45 percent for women and 40 to 50 percent for men.

If we "broke open" a single red blood cell, we would find that it contains about 250 million molecules of hemoglobin (Hb). The hemoglobin molecule is what actually transports oxygen throughout the body. A single molecule of hemoglobin can transport 4 molecules of oxygen. Thus, a single red

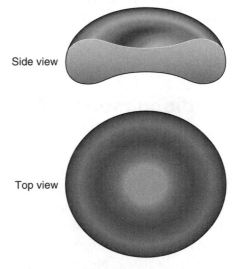

Side view

Top view

Figure 1.9 The structure of a red blood cell.

blood cell (and remember, you have trillions of red blood cells) has the capacity to transport 1 billion molecules of oxygen.

Now that you understand that red blood cells—or more specifically, the hemoglobin molecules contained in red blood cells—transport oxygen throughout the body, let's look at how oxygen-reduced blood becomes oxygen-enriched blood in the lungs. The entire process of oxygen transport is regulated by changes in the partial pressure of oxygen (PO_2) that take place from the moment we inhale air through our nose and mouth until the air reaches our body's tissues and organs. PO_2 decreases as inspired air moves from the nose and mouth to the lungs. The decrease is due to the process of diffusion wherein molecules move from an area of high concentration to an area of low concentration. Specifically, the PO_2 of inspired air at sea level is approximately 159 mm Hg (millimeters of mercury), which drops to 105 mm Hg in the lungs.

As already noted, blood entering the lungs via the pulmonary arteries contains red blood cells that are relatively low in oxygen. The PO_2 of this oxygen-reduced blood is approximately 40 mm Hg. This pressure difference, or pressure gradient, in the lungs (105 mm Hg) compared to the oxygen-reduced blood (40 mm Hg) favors the diffusion of oxygen from the lungs to the oxygen-reduced blood (see figure 1.10), where it binds to hemoglobin molecules. The diffusion of oxygen from the lungs to the blood takes only about 0.75 seconds and occurs across a very sheer membrane in the pulmonary capillaries that is approximately 1/10,000 the width of a Kleenex!

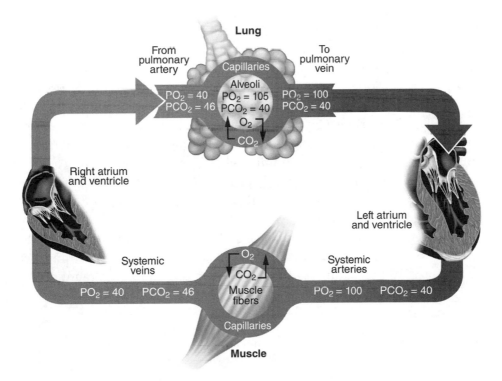

Figure 1.10 Gas exchange between air, lungs, blood, and tissue shows how partial pressure of O_2 and CO_2 drive the exchange.

As a result of the diffusion of oxygen in the lungs, oxygen-enriched blood exits the lungs with a PO$_2$ of 100 mm Hg. The oxygen-enriched blood is transported via the pulmonary veins to the left ventricle of the heart; the blood is then circulated throughout the body, as discussed earlier. When oxygen-enriched blood arrives at the capillary bed of a skeletal muscle, the pressure gradient favors the release of oxygen from hemoglobin to the skeletal muscle. The oxygen-enriched blood is at approximately 100 mm Hg, and the muscle is at about 30 mm Hg. The oxygen that is unloaded in the skeletal muscle can now be used by the mitochondria to produce ATP via the oxidative phosphorylation energy system. Finally, the blood exits the skeletal muscle's capillary bed in an oxygen-reduced state with a PO$_2$ of about 40 mm Hg. The blood returns to the right ventricle of the heart to repeat the process of oxygenation in the lungs and oxygen transport throughout the body.

TRAINING EFFECTS ON THE CARDIOPULMONARY SYSTEM

The ability to transport oxygen efficiently is clearly an important factor contributing to optimal performance in endurance sport, which is heavily dependent on oxidative energy production. Of course, one question that immediately comes to mind among athletes is, "Can I improve my cardiopulmonary system and oxygen transport capabilities through training?" The answer is yes.

One way to improve oxygen transport is to undertake altitude training. This type of training has the effect of increasing the number of red blood cells and hemoglobin molecules, resulting in an increased capacity to get oxygen to the exercising muscles. Many athletes, however, do not have the time or resources to undergo altitude training for a duration that will bring about an increase in red blood cells and hemoglobin. Unfortunately, some unethical athletes have chosen to induce the same physiological effect by using illegal pharmacological ergogenic aids such as recombinant human erythropoietin (rhEPO). Athletes should understand that several positive cardiopulmonary training effects can be acquired at sea level by using a training program that is well designed and scientifically sound.

This section focuses on those beneficial cardiopulmonary training effects. (Chapters 8, 9, 10, and 11 provide specific training programs that help elicit these beneficial cardiopulmonary training effects.) Many cardiopulmonary adaptations occur as a result of regular endurance training. Regular endurance training means a minimum of 30 to 45 minutes per training session and a minimum of 3 to 5 training sessions per week for at least 8 weeks. The beneficial cardiopulmonary adaptations that can occur include the following:

▶ Decrease in resting and exercise heart rate
▶ Increase in total blood volume
▶ Increase in cardiac output

▶ Increase in exercise respiratory capacity

▶ Increase in maximal oxygen uptake ($\dot{V}O_2$max)

▶ Improvement in lactate threshold

▶ Improvement in maximal exercise performance

▶ Improvement in exercise economy

▶ Improvement in endurance performance

▶ Improvement in heat tolerance

▶ Decrease in total body weight

▶ Decrease in body fat

▶ Decrease in blood pressure (if moderate or high blood pressure exists)

The combined effects of the training-induced improvements in cardiac output, maximal oxygen uptake, lactate threshold, exercise economy, and maximal exercise performance clearly have a positive effect on endurance performance. After all, an improvement in performance is what every endurance athlete and coach strives for. However, endurance performance will not improve significantly unless the proper training is done to bring about these beneficial cardiopulmonary training effects. The upcoming sections explore some of these benefits in greater detail.

Heart Rate

Through regular endurance training, the heart becomes stronger via a progressive overload. Because the heart is stronger, it will pump out more blood with each beat. As a result, the heart doesn't have to work as hard, and the person's heart rate at rest and during exercise will be lower than it was before the person began an endurance training program. During exercise, the person's heart rate will be lower at a specific workload. For example, let's say that the person's heart rate taken immediately after running 800 meters on the first day of training was 175 beats per minute (bpm). After 8 weeks of endurance training, the person's heart rate should be significantly lower after running 800 meters at the same pace that the person ran it on the first day of training. The exact amount is difficult to estimate because it varies from person to person.

A person's recovery heart rate will also improve as a result of endurance training. Using the previous example, let's say that it took 3 minutes for the person's heart rate to drop from 175 bpm to 125 bpm after running 800 meters on the first day of training. After 8 weeks of endurance training, the person's heart rate will drop from 175 bpm to 125 bpm in much less than 3 minutes. Again, the improvement in recovery heart rate will vary from person to person. Despite this individual variability, it is safe to say that after a minimum of 8 weeks of endurance training, the person can expect to see improvements in heart rate at rest (lower), heart rate during exercise at the same workload (lower), and heart rate during recovery after a hard effort (less time to recover).

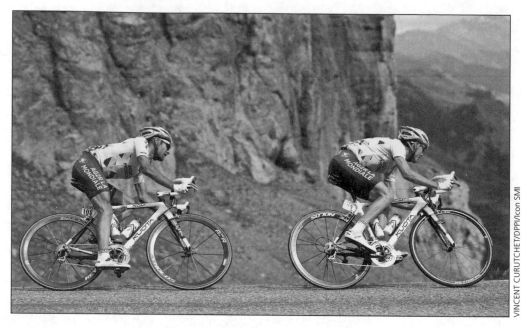

VINCENT CURUTCHET/DPPI/Icon SMI

Well-trained endurance athletes, such has professional cyclists, have a high cardiac output that delivers more oxygen to the muscles.

Cardiac Output

Endurance training also increases the level of a few specific hormones that regulate the amount of blood in the body. These hormones act to increase the fluid portion of the blood, which is called plasma. The overall effect of this hormonal response is an increase in total blood volume. An increase in total blood volume, along with the heart being stronger and more powerful, means that the heart can pump more blood over a specific period of time (at the same heart rate).

This increase in the amount of blood pumped over a specific time is referred to as an increase in cardiac output. Cardiac output is measured as the amount of blood that the heart pumps through the body in a single minute. An increase in cardiac output is important because more blood is delivered to the brain, liver, kidneys, and other important organs. During endurance exercise, an increased cardiac output is important because more blood is delivered to the working skeletal muscles. As a result, more oxygen is delivered to the exercising muscles for energy, whereas carbon dioxide and other metabolic by-products are removed from the exercising muscles more rapidly.

$\dot{V}O_2max$

Endurance training also improves the capacity of the lungs during exercise. This means that the person's respiratory rate (breaths per minute) and tidal volume (liters of air per breath) are improved. These improvements in lung capacity may contribute to an increase in maximal oxygen uptake ($\dot{V}O_2$max). Maximal oxygen uptake is defined as the highest volume of oxygen that a person's body is capable of taking in and using for aerobic energy production. $\dot{V}O_2$max can be expressed in absolute units (liters of oxygen per minute [L × min^{-1}]) or relative units (milliliters of oxygen per kilogram of body mass per minute [ml × kg^{-1} × min^{-1}]). $\dot{V}O_2$max is usually expressed in ml × kg^{-1} × min^{-1} because this value allows us to make comparisons between individuals and tells us who is the fittest "pound for pound."

$\dot{V}O_2$max can rise to levels of 65 to 75 ml × kg^{-1} × min^{-1} and 75 to 85 ml × kg^{-1} × min^{-1} in well-trained female and male endurance athletes, respectively. By comparison, typical values for untrained females and males may range from 35 to 40 ml × kg^{-1} × min^{-1} and 45 to 50 ml × kg^{-1} × min^{-1}, respectively. An improvement in $\dot{V}O_2$max is important because it means that more oxygen is available to the exercising muscles for energy production. Research has shown that a high $\dot{V}O_2$max is one of several physiological factors that contribute to success in endurance sports such as distance running, cross-country skiing, and triathlon.

Lactate Threshold and Maximal Exercise Performance

Scientific research has recently identified a couple of additional physiological factors that are very important contributors to endurance performance: lactate threshold (LT) and maximal exercise performance. These physiological parameters are typically measured under laboratory conditions.

During an increasingly demanding endurance training session or race, the lactate threshold represents the point at which the athlete's body requires a greater contribution from the glycolysis energy system (short-term energy system) and a smaller contribution from the oxidative phosphorylation energy system (long-term energy system). As a result of reaching this point, lactate production exceeds lactate removal, and an exponential increase in blood lactate levels occurs. So, the higher the lactate threshold, the better in terms of endurance performance.

In evaluating lactate threshold capabilities in triathletes, swimming velocity (m × sec^{-1}), cycling power output (watts per kilogram of body weight [W × kg^{-1}]), and running velocity (m × min^{-1}) are the measurements of interest. By participating in a well-designed endurance training program, a triathlete can expect to see significant improvement in these lactate threshold parameters. The athlete will certainly see an improvement in the lactate threshold over the course of a single season. In addition, the athlete will probably see improvements in the lactate threshold from season to season depending on how many years the endurance athlete has been in training.

Maximal exercise performance is simply the objective quantification of an endurance athlete's athletic capability at the point at which the athlete voluntarily stops exercising because of exhaustion (volitional exhaustion). This is determined at the conclusion of a laboratory-based maximal exercise test (e.g., treadmill test).

In evaluating maximal exercise performance in triathletes, the same physiological measurements used for evaluating lactate threshold are of interest, but they are now measured under conditions of maximal effort (instead of lactate threshold effort). Like the lactate threshold, the higher the level of maximal exercise performance, the better in terms of endurance performance. By participating in a well-designed endurance training program, an athlete can expect to see the same type of improvement in maximal exercise performance as seen in the lactate threshold (within a single season and from season to season).

Physiological Economy

Another physiological factor that contributes to endurance performance is economy. The concept of physiological economy is similar to the concept of fuel efficiency in an automobile. We know that a more economical or efficient car uses less gas at a specific speed and gets greater "miles per gallon" than a less economical car. The same is true for endurance athletes.

For example, let's say that athlete A and athlete B both have a similar $\dot{V}O_2$max value of 65 ml $\times$ kg^{-1} $\times$ min^{-1}. However, athlete A uses 50 ml $\times$ kg^{-1} $\times$ min^{-1} while running at a pace of 5 minutes per mile in the first half of a 10K race, whereas athlete B uses 53 ml $\times$ kg^{-1} $\times$ min^{-1} while running at the same pace in the first half of a 10K race. Thus, athlete A is more efficient and economical in terms of energy expenditure than athlete B because he uses less oxygen ("less gas") at the 5-minute-per-mile pace. Athlete A should have a competitive advantage over athlete B in the second half of the race because of his better physiological economy. Several factors can improve physiological economy, including a well-designed endurance training program, individual running biomechanics, uphill running, bungee running, and plyometrics training.

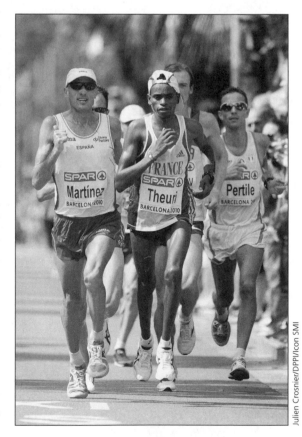

Julien Crosnier/DPPI/Icon SMI

In endurance competitions, having greater physiological economy is essential for success.

Tolerance to Heat and Humidity

A person's ability to work and exercise in heat and humidity is also significantly improved as a result of endurance training. As mentioned earlier, the body produces more plasma and increases the total blood volume when a person performs endurance training on a consistent basis. Think of total blood volume as radiator coolant in a car or truck. Endurance training leads to an increase in total blood volume, which allows a person to have more "radiator coolant" in the body. As a result, the person is able to produce more sweat and dissipate heat more effectively from the body, particularly when exercising in a hot and humid environment. This is a particularly beneficial effect for endurance athletes who often compete in arid or tropical environments.

Body Weight and Body Fat

Endurance training can lower a person's total body weight and reduce body fat. This may not be a major concern for well-trained endurance athletes, because these athletes are typically "lean and mean." However, it may become more important as athletes get older, especially when they reach a point when their lifestyle (job, family, travel, and so on) prevents them from training as they did earlier in their career. For individuals with moderate to high blood pressure, regular endurance training can have a significant lowering effect, thereby decreasing the risk of cardiovascular disease and premature death. Again, this is probably not a major concern for most well-trained endurance athletes, because their blood pressure is typically normal. However, elevated blood pressure may become an issue as an athlete gets older and becomes less active.

SKELETAL MUSCLE CONTRACTION

The physiological process of skeletal muscle contraction is continually operating during our daily activities, even when we are not exercising. Walking up stairs, lifting a book, or even reading this sentence involves skeletal muscle contraction. Of course, the process of skeletal muscle contraction is extremely active during exercise, and it is an important training consideration for people who compete in endurance sport. As described earlier, when ATP is broken down, it provides the energy needed for several physiological functions, including muscular contraction. This section describes the process of skeletal muscle contraction, focusing on the unique anatomical structure of skeletal muscle fiber and the fascinating step-by-step process of muscular contraction.

Similar to the information presented on energy systems, the information on skeletal muscle contraction may seem very technical, but we will sift through some of the irrelevant details and stay focused on the important features of skeletal muscle contraction. Endurance athletes may gain a new appreciation for the intricacies and synchrony of this physiological process. Note: The terms *muscle fiber* and *muscle cell* are used interchangeably in this section.

Skeletal Muscle Anatomy

In describing the anatomy of skeletal muscle, we will move from the general to the specific. Having said that, a good way to think of the anatomical structure of skeletal muscle is to compare it to the cable of a suspension bridge. The cable of a suspension bridge has several internal bundles of smaller-diameter cable wrapped in an overlapping configuration that significantly enhances the strength and stability of the "mother cable." The anatomical structure of skeletal muscle is similar: As we probe deeper into the muscle, the muscle fibers are progressively smaller in diameter and are bundled tightly together; the fibers are reinforced by various connective and overlapping anatomical structures that provide additional support.

Figure 1.11 shows the characteristics of skeletal muscle that are similar to the cable of a suspension bridge. Notice how the muscle fibers get progressively smaller in diameter as you view the figure from upper right to lower left. Also notice the connective and supportive tubelike structures that surround each sequential layer of skeletal muscle. The main structure in the muscle fiber of skeletal muscle is the sarcomere, which lies in the myofibril. The myofibril is very important because it is the basic unit of all skeletal muscle contraction.

A more detailed version of the myofibril and surrounding structures is shown in figure 1.12. Focus on the following important structures that surround the sarcomere: T-tubule, tubules of the sarcoplasmic reticulum, and terminal cisternae of the sarcoplasmic reticulum. These structures are important because they are involved

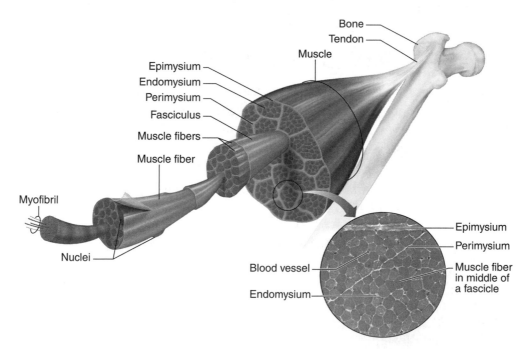

Figure 1.11 Basic structure of skeletal muscle.

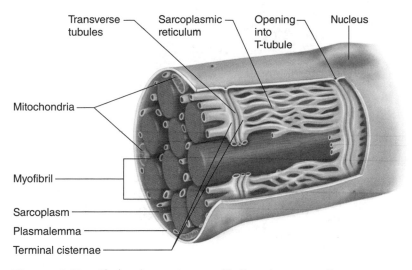

Transverse tubules — Sarcoplasmic reticulum — Opening into T-tubule — Nucleus

Mitochondria —

Myofibril —

Sarcoplasm —

Plasmalemma —

Terminal cisternae —

Figure 1.12 Skeletal muscle: myofibril and surrounding structures.

in the initial phase of skeletal muscle contraction, which is called the excitation phase (described in the next section). Figure 1.12 also shows the mitochondria, which you learned about earlier in this chapter.

Now let's take a detailed look at where the real action of skeletal muscle contraction takes place—the sarcomere. Briefly review the various lines, bands, and zones of the sarcomere shown in figure 1.13 on page 18. The two most important structures in skeletal muscle contraction are actin (thin filament) and myosin (thick filament). The anatomical structure of myosin is shown in the blowup frame on the bottom left. Myosin is made up of a tail segment and two large heads. An important feature of myosin is that the heads have the ability to move. To illustrate this feature, we can compare the structure of myosin to the structure of a person's lower arm: forearm (myosin tail), wrist (joint between myosin tail and heads), and hand (myosin heads). Just as the hand has the ability to flex, extend, and rotate around, so do the myosin heads. This anatomical characteristic is very important in the process of skeletal muscle contraction.

The anatomical structure of actin is shown in the blowup frame on the middle left in figure 1.13. Actin is the double strand of egg-shaped structures lined up in an end-to-end configuration. A thinner protein strand called tropomyosin overlaps the outer surface of actin, and troponin is attached to and positioned at regular intervals on tropomyosin. The bottom half of figure 1.13 shows several actin and myosin filaments in relation to one another. Troponin and tropomyosin are regulatory proteins in a muscle cell, and actin and myosin are contractile proteins. The regulatory proteins help ensure that uncontrolled muscle contractions do not occur, and they prevent uncontrolled binding of actin and myosin.

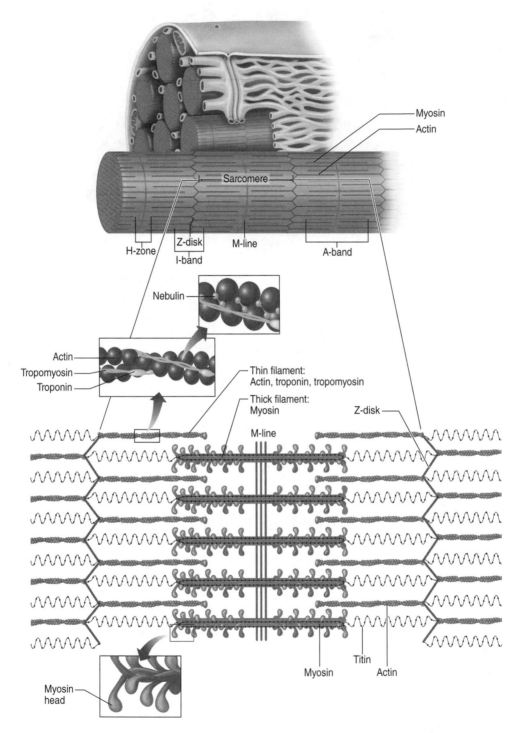

Figure 1.13 Skeletal muscle sarcomere, including the contractile filaments, actin and myosin.

Phases of Skeletal Muscle Contraction

Now that you are familiar with the anatomical structures involved in skeletal muscle contraction, let's look at the sequence of neural, biochemical, and physiological events that allow skeletal muscle contraction to take place. The process of skeletal muscle contraction occurs in three phases (and each of these phases involves several steps):

1. Excitation phase
2. Coupling phase
3. Contraction phase

The excitation phase of muscle contraction (see figure 1.14) refers to the neural impulse that serves to spark the sequence of biochemical and physiological steps that result in skeletal muscle contraction. The key steps in the excitation phase are as follows:

1. Motor nerves embedded in the muscle fire off electrical impulses called action potentials. These action potentials move through the muscle fiber like electricity traveling through a power line (figure 1.14*a*).
2. The action potential moves along the sarcolemma and down the T-tubules to the sarcoplasmic reticulum (figure 1.14*b*).
3. The action potential triggers the release of calcium (Ca^{2+}) from the terminal cisternae of the sarcoplasmic reticulum (figure 1.14*c*).

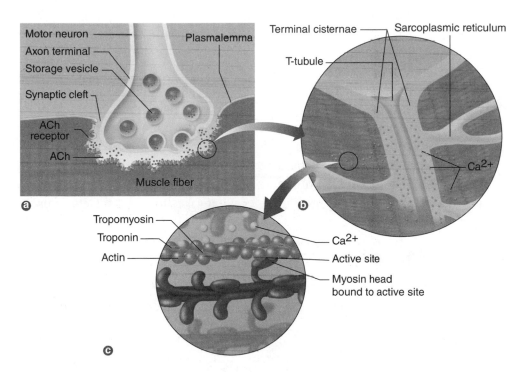

Figure 1.14 The excitation and coupling phases of skeletal muscle contraction.

An interesting side note is how lactic acid affects this process. In the earlier discussion on energy production, you learned that the glycolysis energy system produces two molecules of ATP plus lactic acid, which quickly converts to lactate and H^+ (positively charged hydrogen ions). In addition to other physiological effects, high concentrations of H^+ can obstruct the release of calcium from the terminal cisternae. Essentially, high levels of H^+ serve to gum up the process of skeletal muscle contraction, thereby contributing to premature fatigue.

The coupling phase of skeletal muscle contraction is also shown in figure 1.14 on page 19. Coupling refers to the interconnection of the contractile filaments, actin and myosin. Here are the key steps in the coupling phase:

1. Calcium binds to the troponin complex.
2. The troponin complex changes its shape and configuration, thereby allowing tropomyosin to recede into the space between the actin strands.
3. As tropomyosin recedes from the outer surface of actin, it no longer blocks the outer surface of actin from interfacing with myosin.
4. The binding sites on actin are now fully exposed. The myosin heads quickly attach (couple) to actin at the binding sites.

The contraction phase of skeletal muscle contraction is shown in figure 1.15. Contraction refers to the sequence of events in which myosin essentially "pulls" on actin, thereby drawing the two contractile filaments closer together and resulting in muscular contraction. This phase is usually referred to as the sliding filament theory. Remember that the contraction phase of skeletal muscle contraction will not occur unless ATP is present.

After the contraction phase, the skeletal muscle will return to the relaxed, noncontractile state when the motor nerves stop firing off action potentials, which in turn shuts off the release of calcium from the terminal cisternae of the sarcoplasmic reticulum. Without calcium present, tropomyosin and the troponin complex resume their noncontractile positions—that is, they serve to block myosin from attaching to actin. The process of skeletal muscle contraction is one of the most amazing aspects of human physiology. We hope that you now have a better understanding and appreciation for what takes place in skeletal muscles during endurance activities.

Skeletal Muscle Fiber Types

Traditional textbooks on exercise physiology typically identify three basic types of skeletal muscle fiber in humans. Recent research on animals and humans, however, has provided compelling evidence of several additional pure and hybrid fiber types in skeletal muscle. This research is ongoing, and it is possible that changes in how we classify muscle fibers will occur in the future. For the purpose of this chapter, we focus on the three main skeletal muscle fiber types:

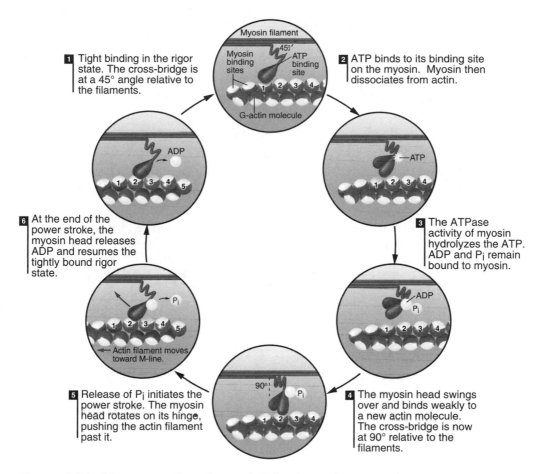

Figure 1.15 The contraction phase of skeletal muscle contraction.

Reprinted, by permission, from W.L. Kenney, J.H. Wilmore, and D.L. Costill, 2012, *Physiology of sport and exercise*, 5th ed. (Champaign, IL: Human Kinetics), 36. Adapted from SILVERTHORN, DEE UN-GLAUB, HUMAN PHYSIOLOGY, 4th, © 2007. Printed and electronically reproduced by permission of Pearson Education, Inc., Upper Saddle River, New Jersey.

▶ Type I: slow oxidative. Type I fibers rely primarily on oxidative phosphorylation for ATP. These fibers typically have a high level of endurance, or the ability to contract repeatedly without fatigue. The soleus muscle in the lower leg is an example of a muscle with many Type I muscle fibers.

▶ Type IIA: fast oxidative glycolytic. Fibers of this type are often considered "tweeners"—that is, they have characteristics of both Type I and Type IIX muscle fibers. The diaphragm muscle contains many Type IIA muscle fibers.

▶ Type IIX: fast glycolytic. Type IIX fibers have the potential to produce a great deal of force, but they also have limited endurance because of their heavy reliance on the short-term energy system for ATP. The gastrocnemius muscle in the lower leg contains many Type IIX muscle fibers.

Most muscles have a certain percentage of Type I, Type IIA, and Type IIX fibers. In other words, the soleus muscle is not made up exclusively of Type I fibers; rather, the soleus has predominantly Type I fibers but also includes lower percentages of Type IIA and Type IIX fibers. Similarly, the diaphragm muscle is predominantly composed of Type IIA fibers, whereas the gastrocnemius muscle is primarily made up of Type IIX fibers.

Type I and Type IIX fibers have very distinct metabolic features. Type I fibers are designed to facilitate oxidative phosphorylation energy production and are found in relative abundance in endurance athletes. In contrast, Type IIX fibers are designed to facilitate glycolytic energy production and are found in relative abundance in sprint and power athletes. Type IIA fibers are essentially a hybrid of Type I and Type IIX fibers and therefore have the capability of producing ATP via oxidative phosphorylation and glycolytic metabolism.

TRAINING EFFECTS ON SKELETAL MUSCLE

Three types of training can alter the physiological and biochemical characteristics of skeletal muscle:

▶ Aerobic (or endurance) training

▶ Anaerobic (or sprint) training

▶ Resistance training

The following sections examine the effects that each of these methods of training have on skeletal muscle.

Aerobic or Endurance Training

Endurance training stresses and challenges Type I (slow oxidative) muscle fibers more than Type IIX (fast glycolytic) muscle fibers. As a result, Type I fibers tend to enlarge with endurance training. Although the percentage of Type I and Type IIX fibers does not appear to change, endurance training may cause Type IIX fibers to take on more of the characteristics of Type IIA (fast oxidative glycolytic) fibers if they are regularly recruited during exercise.

The number of capillaries supplying each muscle fiber increases with endurance training. Recall that the capillary bed is a microscopic, meshlike structure that is embedded deep in the muscle. The capillaries serve as a "transfer point" through which oxygen and nutrients (e.g., glucose) are delivered to the exercising muscles via arterial blood, while carbon dioxide and metabolic by-products (e.g., lactate and positively charged hydrogen ions) are removed via venous blood. This delivery-and-pickup process is enhanced if the number of capillaries is increased, thereby allowing the exercising muscles to perform more efficiently.

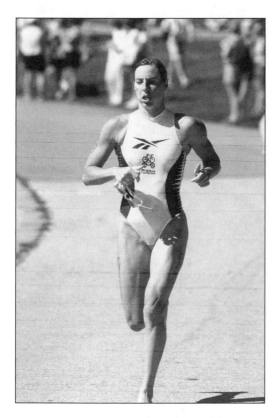

Endurance training leads to several key physiological adaptations that increase an athlete's ability to compete.

Endurance training increases both the number and size of the mitochondria in skeletal muscle. This is particularly true for Type I (slow oxidative) muscle fibers. As described earlier, the mitochondria are microscopic, capsule-shaped units located in the muscle cell (see figures 1.7 on page 5 and 1.13 on page 18) that are essential for the production of ATP via the oxidative phosphorylation energy system (figure 1.6 on page 5). By increasing both the size and number of mitochondria, endurance training enhances oxidative energy production.

The activity of many oxidative enzymes is increased with endurance training. Figure 1.6 is a simplified representation of the oxidative energy system. It shows how 2 molecules of acetyl CoA enter a mitochondrion and move into the Krebs cycle, then on to the electron transport system (ETS) to produce 32 molecules of ATP. The Krebs cycle is a series of biochemical reactions essential to the production of the 32 molecules of ATP, which are ultimately synthesized in the ETS. Most of the oxidative enzymes that are enhanced via endurance training are located in the Krebs cycle phase of the oxidative phosphorylation energy system. Similar to the increase in mitochondria, an increase in the activity of oxidative enzymes serves to enhance oxidative energy production.

Finally, endurance training increases muscle myoglobin content by 75 to 80 percent. Myoglobin is the "smaller brother" of hemoglobin and has many similar structural characteristics. Like hemoglobin, myoglobin's primary physiological function is to transport oxygen. Whereas hemoglobin carries oxygen from the lungs to the exercising muscles via the bloodstream, myoglobin picks up oxygen after it has been dropped off in the capillary bed by hemoglobin. Next, myoglobin transports oxygen to the mitochondria, where the oxygen is used to produce ATP. By increasing myoglobin content, endurance training enhances oxygen delivery within the exercising muscle.

Anaerobic or Sprint Training

Anaerobic training increases ATP-CP and glycolytic enzymes in skeletal muscle. Some of these enzymes are shown in figure 1.4 (immediate energy system; on page 3) and 1.5 (short-term energy system; on page 4). Similar to the increase in the oxidative enzymes, increases in the ATP-CP and glycolytic enzymes will serve to enhance the production of ATP by those two energy systems.

Another benefit of anaerobic training is that it can increase the buffering capacity of skeletal muscle. As described earlier, lactate and positively charged hydrogen ions (H^+) are metabolites that are produced in the glycolysis energy system. High concentrations of H^+ can slow down the release of calcium (Ca^{2+}) in the excitation phase of skeletal muscle contraction, thereby contributing to premature fatigue of the muscle. As a result of anaerobic training, the amount of bicarbonate (HCO_3^-) in skeletal muscle is increased. As shown in figure 1.16, bicarbonate acts as a very effective buffer for reducing acidosis in the exercising muscle. Bicarbonate essentially picks up the potentially detrimental H^+ and subsequently removes it safely from the body in the form of H_2O and CO_2.

$$C_3H_5O_8^- + H^+ + HCO_3^- \longrightarrow H_2CO_3 \longrightarrow H_2O + CO_2$$
$$\text{Lactate} \qquad \text{Bicarbonate}$$

Figure 1.16 Equation showing bicarbonate buffering to reduce acidosis in exercising muscle.

Resistance Training

Athletes may use various types of resistance training programs (e.g., heavy weight and low reps versus moderate weight and high reps), and many physiological adaptations occur as a result of regular resistance training. Regular resistance training means a minimum of 3 to 5 training sessions per week for at least 8 weeks.

An increase in the actual size of the skeletal muscle fiber is known as hypertrophy. Most research studies have shown that regular resistance training in combination with an adequate diet will produce skeletal muscle hypertrophy. The degree of hypertrophy will vary depending on the specific resistance training program (weight, reps, number of training sessions per week, and so on).

Regular resistance training also increases the number of muscle motor units that are active. A single muscle motor unit is made up of several muscle fibers along with the nerve that innervates those muscle fibers and stimulates them to contract in unison. To better understand how muscle motor units work, just think of a group of 10 athletes pulling on a rope tied to a car. Each individual athlete can be compared to an individual muscle motor unit. (In this case, the term *motor* refers to movement, not the motor of the car.) If all 10 athletes are pulling hard on the rope, this represents a much stronger "muscle" than if only 5 of the 10 athletes are pulling on it because there are twice as many "active muscle motor units." The same is true in relation to resistance training. After several weeks of resistance training, the skeletal muscle has produced more active motor units (or people pulling on the rope) than there were before the person started the resistance training program.

Muscular strength is increased as a result of resistance training. Muscular strength is defined as the maximum force that is generated by a muscle or muscle group. Muscular strength is usually measured using a one-repetition maximum (1RM) lift, or the maximum amount of weight that an individual can lift just once. An athlete who can bench press 300 pounds in a 1RM has twice the muscular strength as an athlete who can bench press 150 pounds in a 1RM.

Resistance training also increases muscular power, which is not the same as muscular strength. Muscular power is the explosive aspect of strength and is the product of muscular strength and the speed of a specific movement. For example, athlete A and athlete B can both bench press 150 pounds in a 1RM. However, athlete A completes the lift in 1 second whereas athlete B can complete the lift in 1/2 of a second. Although athlete B has the same muscular strength as athlete A, he has twice the muscular power because he can lift the same weight in half the time.

Muscular endurance is another important performance characteristic for endurance athletes, and this characteristic is also enhanced via regular resistance training. Muscular endurance refers to the capacity to sustain repeated muscular actions, such as when running for an extended period of time. It also refers to the ability to sustain fixed or static muscular actions for an extended period of time, such as when attempting to pin an opponent in wrestling. Muscular endurance is usually measured by counting the number of repetitions that an athlete can perform at a fixed percentage of the athlete's 1RM. For example, if the athlete bench presses 200 pounds in a 1RM, the athlete's muscular endurance can be measured by counting how many repetitions the athlete can complete at 75 percent of the 1RM (150 pounds).

CHAPTER 2

Endurance Tests and Assessments

Neal Henderson
Will Kirousis
Jason Gootman

Training programs are traditionally used by competitive athletes to maximize training effectiveness and performance improvement. However, any well-designed training program can also be useful for noncompetitive and recreational athletes, allowing these athletes to maximize enjoyment and minimize the risk of injury or overtraining. To measure the effectiveness of an endurance training program, regular testing should be done. The testing may be performed in a laboratory setting, but field testing is usually more convenient for both the coach and the athletes. Ideally, testing should include measures for movement analysis, aerobic endurance, and muscle endurance. This chapter reviews some common testing protocols and the methods used to analyze the data collected during the testing sessions.

Testing for the sake of testing will not provide any guidance for a coach or athlete. For any tests conducted, the information gathered should be used to provide feedback to the athlete. Too often coaches and exercise physiologists ask athletes to perform extremely taxing tests and evaluations but fail to effectively communicate the results of those tests to the athlete. The information gained in testing sessions needs to be shared with the athlete in a timely manner and then used to guide changes in training.

Before conducting any testing, the coach needs to properly calibrate any testing equipment. All equipment used for testing should be maintained and calibrated according to the manufacturer's recommendations. Testing conducted with equipment that is not calibrated or is incorrectly calibrated will result in data that are not valid or reliable. If the analysis of a training program's effectiveness is based on data that are not valid or reliable, then the analysis will be flawed.

MOVEMENT ANALYSIS AND BIOMECHANICS

Endurance sports are typically not thought of as highly technical endeavors (unlike sports such as golf, baseball, and tennis), but proper movement during training and competition for endurance sports can affect both performance and health. The study of biomechanics refers to analyzing human motion with regard to physics, kinematics, and mechanics. Most endurance sport movements are repeated hundreds or thousands of times each training session. Therefore, proper mechanics are critical to an endurance athlete's ability to optimize performance and avoid injury. Movement evaluation can be performed using a well-trained eye, video capture, a computer, or specialized biomechanics equipment—such as pressure sensors, force plates, and three-dimensional computer motion analysis programs (see figure 2.1).

Every endurance athlete has a unique physical build as well as strengths, weaknesses, and asymmetries that will dictate personal movement style; however, within each sport, some general movement patterns are more effective and are considered proper form. For example, during running, the foot should land nearly underneath the knee to reduce braking movement on each stride and to reduce the stress placed on the musculoskeletal system. When cycling, the knee and foot should travel in a vertical path, overlapping one another when viewed from the front. This reduces stress on the knee joint. When swimming, proper mechanics will allow the athlete to move through the water more easily by producing less drag and will also reduce strain on the shoulder joint.

Coaches and athletes can learn to analyze motion by viewing

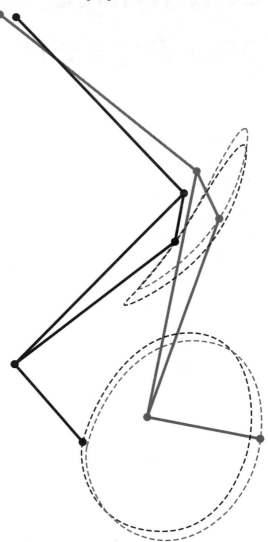

Figure 2.1 This image represents three-dimensional data of a cyclist's pedal stroke. The round tracings are the tracking of the toe, and the ellipses are the paths that the kneecaps travel. The black line represents the right leg, and the gray line represents the left leg.

performances of the proper form and mechanics within their sport. They can do this in person or by reviewing video. Keep in mind that the top athletes in a given sport do not always use optimal biomechanics and may be successful despite their technique. Variations from one athlete to another are normal, but coaches should be able to evaluate an athlete's biomechanics and suggest drills and corrections that will help the athlete improve. Coaches often use video to record their athletes' techniques. Video analysis can be used to slow the body movements to a speed that allows viewers to discern small details that the unaided eye might not see. Coaches should review the video with their athletes to reinforce effective movement patterns and point out areas for improvement.

Athletes who do not have a personal coach can do much of this evaluation by themselves or with the help of a partner who can run the video camera or digital camera. Free or low-cost video analysis programs often come standard on a computer. However, more technical software packages such as Dartfish technology allow for more comprehensive video analysis (including synchronizing multiple camera views, drawing angles, and adding comments or written text on videos).

More sophisticated equipment such as pressure sensors and three-dimensional imaging systems may be available at specialized sports medicine facilities, medical facilities, universities, and other research institutions. These tools can be used by biomechanists and specially trained clinical staff to take a closer look at the movements an athlete is making. Many endurance athletes and coaches overlook the use of biomechanical analysis as a tool for helping to modify or improve an athlete's current mechanics. The typical thinking is that endurance athletes move the way that they naturally do and should just improve their fitness without worrying about poor mechanics. Although the differences in improved mechanics can be subtle, they are very effective in reducing injury and improving performance.

Movement analysis can also help determine the types of sport-specific and supplemental training, such as resistance training, that can improve performance. Proper analysis should include evaluation of the actual muscle groups being used (prime movers and stabilizers), the type of muscle action occurring (concentric, eccentric, isometric, or a combination of these), the velocity of contraction and movement, the range of motion of the joints, and the type of energy system used to deliver energy (immediate, short-term, or long-term energy system). All of these factors should be known before prescribing training and exercises meant to improve an individual's capability and performance.

Figure 2.2 presents a worksheet that athletes can use to perform their own movement analysis. An athlete should complete this form periodically to monitor movement changes and adaptations that can occur with regular training. The best strategy is to complete the form every 4 to 8 weeks after completing similar workouts. The form is subjective and can be used for any sport or activity, but it works best for those activities that are repetitive—such as running, biking, and swimming.

Figure 2.2   Movement Analysis Worksheet

Athlete's name: _____   Date: _____

Sport: _____   Location: _____

GENERAL IMPRESSION

_____

_____

_____

_____

_____

SPECIFIC OBSERVATIONS

Range of motion:_____

_____

Symmetry and asymmetry: _____

_____

Coordination of movement: _____

_____

Timing and rhythm: _____

_____

ADDITIONAL NOTES

_____

_____

_____

_____

_____

_____

From NSCA, 2012, *Developing endurance* (Champaign, IL: Human Kinetics).

FIELD TESTING

Evaluating an athlete's progress outside of actual competition helps determine how to adjust training loads, and it provides important feedback to the athlete during extended periods of training. In addition, some athletes do not compete in events or only compete a limited number of times each year. For these athletes, routine testing helps ensure that the training they are performing is improving their fitness and their performance potential.

Another reason to include testing in the training schedule is to build athletes' confidence. Evaluating the changes in performance from one training cycle to another is one of the simplest ways for athletes to gain a mental edge when they compete. Consistent testing can measure performance improvement, which helps keep motivation high. If athletes see improvement, they will be more convinced that the training program is working. Evidence of improvement can also motivate athletes who are not competing regularly. In addition, comparisons can be performed in order to track fitness and performance levels from season to season and from year to year. In endurance sports, it typically takes many years of dedicated training for athletes to reach their full potential. Initially, the gains are larger, but they tend to decrease over time.

Laboratory tests are ideal for objectively evaluating markers of fitness, but field tests can be done more frequently and allow more sport-specific adaptations to be evaluated. Also, athletes often feel more comfortable with field tests because the tests take place in the athletes' natural element. If possible, though, field testing should be a replication of lab-based testing—but with a change in the setting. Field tests can be performed at specific time intervals during a training schedule as a way to track progress; they can also be conducted to practice pacing strategies, nutrition strategies, new equipment, and other areas that the athlete needs to experiment with before competition.

Testing Guidelines

When possible, field tests should be conducted in the environment where the athlete competes. For example, a triathlete may want to evaluate swimming, cycling, and running progress at the end of each rest cycle (typically every 3 to 6 weeks). For the swim, most triathlon competitions occur in open water, such as a lake or ocean; however, finding a suitable location with a known distance may not be feasible, especially at certain times of the year. In this case, the test can be performed in a swimming pool.

The ideal field test would be between one-third of the race distance and the full race distance. For example, a 1,500-meter swim is standard for an athlete preparing for a triathlon. Field tests may also be conducted at a constrained performance level (based on heart rate or perceived effort) for a given distance or time. Depending on the race focus, field tests may be as short as 5 seconds or as long as 1 hour. To ensure repeatability in retests, note the number of rest days taken before the field test, the warm-up procedures, the nutrition intake before and during the test, and any other factors that may influence future tests.

Each field test should be performed under similar, if not exact, conditions. One aspect of the conditions is the course used to conduct the test. A set course should usually be used when performing the field tests. Having a set course is especially important when testing athletes in sports such as rowing or cross-country skiing, where water and snow conditions may vary. Environmental conditions must also be considered when testing cyclists; for these athletes, a route should be selected that is not subject to dramatic variations in wind.

Another aspect of testing conditions is the effort level of the athlete. Although all-out efforts might seem to be the best reflection of improvements in fitness, they are not always the best option. An athlete may find it difficult to get motivated to perform a maximal effort outside of actual competition. And if the athlete's motivation on test day is not high, the athlete may underachieve, even when the athlete's fitness has improved compared to previous field tests. Therefore, field tests are often more valid when conducted at a predetermined submaximal effort. This also helps ensure that the effort can be repeated more reliably in future tests. In addition, unique characteristics of the various types of athletes need to be considered when determining how to conduct a field test.

Tools such as wireless heart rate monitors and GPS units allow athletes to track speed and heart rate and then download these data for further analysis after the performance. Using a portable power meter on a bicycle is a very effective way to evaluate the power sustained during field tests. A chief advantage of using these tools is that they provide excellent information that can be compared season after season.

Testing Types and Intensity Levels

Another important consideration is how to classify exercise intensity in workouts. Using time trials in field tests is a very practical way to gauge the current ability level of athletes and to determine personalized intensity zones. These tests are convenient and inexpensive, and they are similar to what athletes experience in workouts and races; thus, they provide very useful information. Time-trial field tests (such as the ones on pages 34 through 38) are races against the clock that allow athletes to record various forms of intensity data. Table 2.1 suggests which tests various endurance athletes should perform. Tests should be performed at the beginning of a training year and then every 12 to 20 weeks.

Once testing is complete, an athlete's intensity zones can be determined. Here are the four intensities:

1. Easy intensity
2. Aerobic intensity
3. Anaerobic intensity
4. Race intensity

Table 2.1 Recommended Testing for Various Endurance Athletes

Type of athlete	Recommended tests
Triathlete	Swimming test, cycling tests, running test
Off-road triathlete	Swimming test, cycling tests, running test
Duathlete	Cycling tests, running test
Off-road duathlete	Cycling tests, running test
Cyclist	Cycling tests
Mountain bike racer	Cycling tests
Runner	Running test

No calculations are necessary to determine an athlete's easy intensity zones. Table 2.2 shows recommended ratings of perceived exertion that can be used to help athletes understand what easy intensity should feel like. In short, easy intensity is similar to the effort level used when walking. The descriptions refer to the level of difficulty in breathing. A rating of 1 or "extremely easy" is what it feels like to breathe when walking at a leisurely pace. A rating of 10 or "extremely hard" is what it feels like to breathe at the end of a short race (e.g., a 5K) or at the end of a $\dot{V}O_2$ max test. For an athlete's easy zone, the intensity should be at a rating of between 1 and 3. Perceived exertion is the best way to monitor the easy intensity zone.

Perceived exertion can also be used for the more intense zones; however, more precise measures work better. The tables accompanying the following time-trial tests show what measurements (average speeds or paces, power outputs, or heart rates from an athlete's time-trial field tests) are used to determine the intensity zones.

Table 2.2 Ratings of Perceived Exertion

Rating	Description
1	Extremely easy
2	Very easy
3	Easy
4	
5	Moderately hard
6	
7	Hard
8	
9	Very hard
10	Extremely hard

CYCLING TESTS

Outdoor Test: 10-Mile Time Trial

Equipment

Power meter or cycling computer and heart rate monitor

Course Selection

Select a course that is safe and free of anything that would require riders to stop (e.g., traffic lights, poor road conditions). Be sure the course is one that can be used to complete additional tests in the future for comparison.

Procedure

1. Athletes warm up by riding for 15 minutes. They ride the last 3 minutes at their projected test intensity. They should finish the warm-up at the location where they will begin the 10-mile time trial.
2. Athletes ride easy for 2 minutes.
3. Athletes ride a 10-mile time trial, covering the 10 miles as fast as they can.
4. If using a power meter, athletes note their average power output for the 10 miles.
5. From the power meter or heart rate monitor, athletes note their average heart rate for the 10 miles.
6. From the cycling computer or power meter, athletes note their average speed for the 10 miles.
7. Athletes note their test scores. The test score includes the athlete's average power output (if using a power meter), average heart rate, and average speed (e.g., 211 watts, 162 bpm, and 21.3 mph).
8. After the time trial, athletes ride very easy for 10 to 15 minutes to cool down.

Indoor Test: 30-Minute Time Trial

Equipment

Power meter or cycling computer that measures distance via rear wheel pickup and heart rate monitor

Test Setup

Athletes perform this test on an indoor trainer.

Procedure

1. Athletes warm up by riding for 15 minutes. They ride the last 3 minutes at their projected test intensity.
2. Athletes ride easy for 2 minutes.
3. Athletes ride a 30-minute time trial, going as hard as they can for 30 minutes.
4. If using a power meter, athletes note their average power output for the 30 minutes.
5. From the power meter or heart rate monitor, athletes note their average heart rate for the 30 minutes.
6. Athletes note their test scores. The test score includes the athlete's average power output (if using a power meter) and average heart rate (e.g., 191 watts, 157 bpm).
7. After the time trial, athletes ride very easy for 10 to 15 minutes to cool down.

Percentages Used to Determine Intensity Zones

Intensity level	% of average power output (watts)	% of average heart rate (bpm)	% of average speed (mph)
Easy intensity (EZ)	–	–	–
Aerobic intensity (A)	65-75	77-83	75-85
Anaerobic intensity (AN)	95-105	97-103	95-105
Anaerobic intensity for hill workouts and big-gear workouts (AN H)	105-115	97-103	–
Race intensity for a sprint-distance triathlon (SDT R)	97-107	98-104	97-107
Race intensity for an Olympic-distance triathlon (ODT R)	87-97	92-98	92-102
Race intensity for a half Ironman (1/2 IM R)	77-87	86-92	85-95
Race intensity for an Ironman (IM R)	67-77	80-86	76-86

RUNNING THREE-MILE TIME TRIAL

Equipment

Pace monitor or GPS (optional) and heart rate monitor

Course Selection

Select a three-mile course that is safe and free of anything that would require runners to stop. Be sure to select a course that can be used to complete additional tests in the future for comparison. This test can be performed on a track. If the test is done on a track, the runner should run on the inside lane. The test may also be performed on a treadmill; in that case, the treadmill should be set at a 1 percent incline.

Procedure

1. Athletes warm up by running for 15 minutes. They run the last 2 minutes at their projected test intensity. They should finish the warm-up at the location where they will begin the three-mile time trial.

2. The athletes walk for 2 minutes.

3. Athletes run a three-mile time trial, covering the three miles as fast as they can.

4. If using a pace monitor, athletes note their average pace for the three miles. If not using a pace monitor, athletes should note their time for the three miles and calculate their pace in minutes per mile. For example, if an athlete ran the three miles in 21:30, the athlete's pace in minutes per mile equals 21:30 divided by 3, which is 7:10 per mile.

5. From the pace monitor or heart rate monitor, athletes note their average heart rate for the three miles.

6. Athletes note their test scores. The test score includes the athlete's average pace and average heart rate (e.g., 7:10 per mile, 173 bpm).

7. After the time trial, athletes walk for 10 to 15 minutes to cool down.

Percentages Used to Determine Intensity Zones

Intensity level	% of average pace (min per mile)	% of average heart rate (bpm)
Easy intensity (EZ)	–	–
Aerobic intensity (A)	80-90	77-83
Anaerobic intensity (AN)	95-105	97-103
Race intensity for a 5K (5K R)	97-102	98-104
Race intensity for a 10K (10K R)	92-97	92-98
Race intensity for a half marathon (1/2 Marathon R)	87-92	86-92
Race intensity for a marathon (Marathon R)	82-87	80-86
Race intensity for a sprint-distance triathlon (SDT R)	92-97	97-107
Race intensity for an Olympic-distance triathlon (ODT R)	86-91	–
Race intensity for a half Ironman (1/2 IM R)	80-85	–
Race intensity for an Ironman (IM R)	74-79	–

SWIMMING 500-YARD TIME TRIAL

Equipment

Heart rate monitor (optional)

Procedure

1. Athletes warm up by swimming for 10 minutes. They swim the last 2 minutes at their projected test intensity.
2. The athletes rest for 1 minute.
3. The athletes swim a 500-yard time trial, covering the 500 yards as fast as they can.
4. Athletes note their time for the 500 yards and calculate their pace in minutes per 100 yards (e.g., 1:45 per 100 yards).
5. If athletes can wear a heart rate monitor while swimming, they should record their average heart rate for the 500 yards. If they cannot wear a heart rate monitor, they should take their carotid or radial pulse for 10 seconds immediately after finishing the 500 yards. They can multiply the 10-second pulse by 6 to estimate their heart rate in beats per minute (e.g., 24 beats × 6 = 144 bpm).
6. Athletes note their test scores. The test score includes the athlete's average pace and average heart rate (e.g., 1:45 per 100 yards, 144 bpm).
7. After the time trial, athletes should swim very easy for 5 to 10 minutes to cool down.

Percentages Used to Determine Intensity Zones

Intensity level	% of average 100-yd pace	% of average heart rate (bpm)
Easy intensity (EZ)	–	–
Aerobic intensity (A)	85-95	77-83
Anaerobic intensity (AN)	95-105	97-103
Race intensity for a sprint-distance triathlon (SDT R)	97-107	98-104
Race intensity for an Olympic-distance triathlon (ODT R)	93.5-105	92-98
Race intensity for a half Ironman (1/2 IM R)	90-100	86-92
Race intensity for an Ironman (IM R)	86.5-96.5	80-86

Consider a runner training for a half marathon who completed the running time-trial test in 21:30 for an example of using the time trial to determine intensity levels. To determine this athlete's pace in minutes per mile, divide 21:30 by 3. The result is 7:10 per mile. Table 2.3 provides the calculations for determining this athlete's intensity ranges. Athletes can use their own results (pace per mile) from the three-mile test to calculate their own intensity ranges.

Table 2.3 Intensity Range Calculations (Using Pace) for a Half Marathoner

Intensity	% of pace	Calculation (pace in sec)*	Target training pace (in sec)	Target training pace (in min and sec)
Bottom of aerobic intensity range	80%	430/0.80	538	8:58
Top of aerobic intensity range	90%	430/0.90	478	7:58
Aerobic intensity range				**8:58-7:58 per mile**
Bottom of anaerobic intensity range	95%	430/0.95	453	7:33
Top of anaerobic intensity range	105%	430/1.05	410	6:50
Anaerobic intensity range				**7:33-6:50 per mile**
Bottom of race intensity range for a half marathon	87%	430/0.87	494	8:14
Top of race intensity range for a half marathon	92%	430/0.92	467	7:47
Race intensity range for a half marathon				**8:14-7:47 per mile**

*430 seconds is a pace of 7:10 minutes per mile.

Athletes only need to calculate the race intensity for the distance of the races that they are training for. A spreadsheet can be used to quickly calculate athletes' intensity zones using these formulas. For swimming and running, pace is the best measure of intensity, followed by heart rate. For cycling, power output is the best measure, followed by heart rate. The intensity ranges based on heart rate can be calculated in the same fashion as described for pace. However, separate training zones need to be calculated for each sport. If an athlete takes the running test and attempts to use the resulting HR training zones for cycling, the intensity may be too great. Each time the athletes are tested, which should be done every 12 to 20 weeks, intensity zones can be adjusted.

When doing a set of intervals at anaerobic intensity, athletes should start the set at the low end of their anaerobic intensity zone. As they get into the set, if they can go harder than that, they should do so. However, athletes need to pace themselves. The goal is to complete the whole set, and athletes should try to finish as strong as or stronger than they started. Table 2.4 shows an example of an effective pace strategy for a set of swimming intervals (10 × 100 yards) at anaerobic intensity; the strategy shown in this example is for an athlete with an anaerobic intensity zone for swimming of 1:40 to 1:32 per 100 yards.

Athletes must avoid going too hard early on and having to struggle to finish the set at a lower intensity. Posting a fast time on the first interval or two may be an ego boost, but it's not the best way to maximize potential training benefits. Table 2.5 provides an example of poorly paced intervals. This example is a useful tool for instructing athletes what not to do.

Table 2.4 Well-Paced Intervals

Work interval 1	1:40
Work interval 2	1:38
Work interval 3	1:38
Work interval 4	1:37
Work interval 5	1:38
Work interval 6	1:36
Work interval 7	1:36
Work interval 8	1:34
Work interval 9	1:34
Work interval 10	1:33

Table 2.5 Poorly Paced Intervals

Work interval 1	1:25
Work interval 2	1:28
Work interval 3	1:35
Work interval 4	1:35
Work interval 5	1:37
Work interval 6	1:35
Work interval 7	1:40
Work interval 8	1:45
Work interval 9	1:46
Work interval 10	1:50

AEROBIC ENDURANCE MEASURES AND ANALYSES

During most endurance competitions, athletes rely heavily on energy developed through the aerobic system. For this reason, the training plans for many endurance athletes place almost exclusive focus on the development of aerobic fitness and endurance. The VO_2max test is the most effective measurement of the body's ability to deliver and use oxygen for producing energy that can be used by the muscles. VO_2max (also known as maximum aerobic power) simply stands for the maximal volume of oxygen (O_2) that can be used.

This measurement is important because the more oxygen an individual can consume, the more energy (ATP) can be produced for the muscles to use to contract. For the athlete to move faster, more energy must be available to enable a muscle to contract more rapidly, contract with more force, or some combination of these two. Therefore, the more energy an athlete can liberate through the aerobic system, the faster the athlete can move.

Measurement of this variable requires the use of devices that measure oxygen and carbon dioxide along with a monitor of breathing volume and rate. The process involves measuring the amount of oxygen consumed with each breath, the amount of carbon dioxide produced by the athlete, and the amount of air that the athlete is breathing in and out. All of these measures are used to calculate the actual extraction of oxygen from ambient air for use by the muscles to generate usable energy.

Keep in mind the basic calculations that are used to derive oxygen consumption values. Basically, oxygen consumption ($\dot{V}O_2$) is equal to cardiac output multiplied by the difference in arterial and venous blood oxygen (A-V O_2 difference) concentrations. This is expressed by the following equation:

$$\dot{V}O_2 = \text{cardiac output (Q)} \times \text{(A-V) } O_2 \text{ difference}$$

Cardiac output is determined by the following:

$$\text{Cardiac output} = \text{heart rate} \times \text{stroke volume}$$

Therefore, oxygen consumption can also be expressed this way:

$$\dot{V}O_2 = \text{heart rate} \times \text{stroke volume} \times \text{(A-V) } O_2 \text{ difference}$$

As exercise intensity increases, cardiac output rises, and extraction of oxygen from the blood by the muscles increases. This results in increasing $\dot{V}O_2$. At some point, maximal heart rate (and therefore, cardiac output) is achieved, and $\dot{V}O_2$ plateaus with increasing work rate. The highest rate of oxygen consumption measured is typically defined as $\dot{V}O_2$max.

A typical $\dot{V}O_2$max test begins with a warm-up of 10 to 15 minutes of relatively easy effort followed by a progressive test to exhaustion. The progressive portion of the test should take between 6 and 12 minutes depending on when the athlete reaches fatigue. Typical cutoff points for a $\dot{V}O_2$max test include reaching volitional fatigue, reaching a plateau in $\dot{V}O_2$ with increasing work rate, and reaching a respiratory quotient ($\dot{V}CO_2/\dot{V}O_2$) greater than 1.10. The test data gathered during a $\dot{V}O_2$max test may include the measurement of the ventilatory threshold (VT) as identified by characteristic changes in respiration rate (V_E) versus $\dot{V}O_2$. The ventilatory equivalents of O_2 and CO_2 ($\dot{V}CO_2$ and $\dot{V}O_2$) versus V_E may also be plotted to identify the ventilatory threshold.

The ventilatory threshold is typically used to identify the maximum sustainable effort that an athlete can maintain. It is often correlated to the lactate threshold, which is identified by measuring blood lactate concentrations during progressive exercise testing. The definition of the lactate threshold point varies from lab to lab and from one physiologist or coach to another; however, as long as consistent methods are used to identify the threshold, comparisons from one test to another can be made. Other factors to consider when comparing test data from one lab to another include the elevation of the test facility, the length of the stages used, the increases in work rate from one stage to another, the warm-up protocol, the pretest nutrition and hydration instructions, and the amount of rest before the testing.

Measurement of oxygen consumption via indirect calorimetry (oxygen uptake) can also be used to calculate energy expenditure during exercise. These calculations can determine the total calories of energy oxidized as well as the percentages and amount of carbohydrate and fat being used at each workload. This kind of analysis is very helpful for athletes who want to calculate actual energy expenditure in order to monitor nutrition intake (e.g., athletes with goals for body composition). These data are also helpful for athletes competing in long-distance events where glycogen stores are likely to be depleted during competition; these athletes can use the information to devise appropriate fueling and pacing strategies. The best scenario is when an exercise physiologist and a registered dietitian (one who has sport nutrition experience) can work together to present these data to athletes and help them devise proper nutrition goals.

Lactate profile testing can be performed with or without oxygen consumption or indirect calorimetry measurements. As previously mentioned, the method used to determine the threshold point is less important than using a consistent testing protocol. The lab at the Boulder Center for Sports Medicine (where Neal Henderson works) has performed thousands of lactate profile and $\dot{V}O_2$max tests on all levels of athletes. These athletes have included NHL ice hockey teams, Olympic cyclists and triathletes, recreational runners, and individuals with cardiovascular and pulmonary disease. The researchers at this facility have found that good results are provided when the testing method involves using 4-minute stages, starting at a level that allows for seven to nine stages of progressive intensity, and monitoring heart rate, rating of perceived exertion (RPE), and blood lactate at each stage. In addition, the quality of the lactate-measuring device cannot be overlooked, and daily calibration and proper maintenance help ensure consistent results.

Figure 2.3 provides the lactate profile of a professional cyclist tested at the start of the season. All stages were 4 minutes long. The top line being plotted is heart rate (right vertical axis), and the bottom line is lactate level (left vertical axis). Heart rate is linear as workload increases. In other words, there is a direct relationship between heart rate and workload. Lactate level increases in a linear manner as workload increases until the seventh stage; at that point, a sharp upturn or increase in lactate occurs, indicating lactate threshold. The goal of training is to move the upturn to the right on the graph—that is, the goal is for lactate threshold to occur at a higher workload.

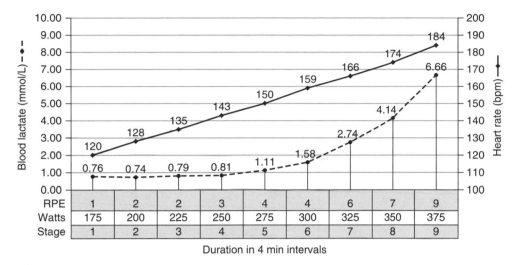

Threshold data		Prescribed training zones					
		By power output (watts)		By perceived effort (RPE)		By heart rate (bpm)	
Power output (watts):	325	Zone 1	<175	Zone 1	<1	Zone 1	<120
Heart rate at LT:	166	Zone 2	175-250	Zone 2	1-3	Zone 2	120-143
Percent of peak heart rate (194)	86%	Zone 3	250-320	Zone 3	3-5	Zone 3	143-164
Mass (kg):	67.3	Zone 4	325-370	Zone 4	6-8	Zone 4	166-180
Power/weight ratio (watts/kg):	4.83	Zone 5	>375	Zone 5	>8	Zone 5	>180

Normal blood lactate resting range: 0.7-2.1 mmol/L

Figure 2.3 Lactate profile of a professional cyclist.

IMPLICATIONS OF ENDURANCE TEST RESULTS

Determining training zones is a common reason for performing testing with athletes. Coaches and athletes use a variety of methods to categorize training zones. Coaches must ensure that their athletes have a clear understanding of the zones used in their training programs. This will help prevent confusion if athletes compare training programs with other athletes or if they read about training programs or recommendations in magazines. For example, for training programs created at the Boulder Center for Sports Medicine, training zones are defined using heart rate ranges, RPE ranges, and power or pace ranges. This method provides multiple reference points that the athletes can use to evaluate how hard they are working. Because multiple formats are provided, athletes can choose the method that is most convenient or helpful to them.

This text includes chapters that cover specific training programming. In each of these chapters, the training zones used in the programs are identified so that the coach and athlete will have a clear understanding of how training intensities are defined. This will go a long way toward reducing confusion and misunderstanding about program execution.

Each method of measuring training intensity has advantages and disadvantages. Athletes and coaches will want to determine which method works best for each individual athlete. Whatever method is chosen, the important thing is that the athlete and coach can communicate using a common terminology. This will help ensure that both the coach and the athlete understand the goals and expectations for the training program.

CHAPTER 3

Endurance Training Principles and Considerations

Bob Seebohar
Ben Reuter

One of the primary goals of a well-designed endurance training program is to help the athlete achieve positive physiological adaptations through proper training and recovery so that the athlete can optimally peak for competition. A well-designed program will also reduce the chance of injury and illness while promoting systematic recovery throughout the training plan. When an athlete experiences a high training load, the body is placed under a great deal of physiological stress. The body does not begin to positively adapt to that stress until proper recovery takes place. A common error is believing that more is always better when it comes to endurance training. However, training without adequate recovery leads to overtraining (often referred to as underrecovery), illness, and burnout. In contrast, too much recovery without training can lead to a deconditioned state or lack of preparation. The amount and timing of both training and recovery are very important when designing a training program for endurance athletes.

DESIGN AND PLANNING

Recovery-based training should be a primary focus of program design. Without adequate recovery, athletes will not optimally progress and reach their full potential. Note that recovery does not only mean days of rest without activity. Recovery takes many forms, including things such as skill and technique practice, massage, good sleep, aerobic cross-training, and proper nutrition. All of these are important in implementing recovery within a training program. Designing a training program for endurance athletes requires four steps:

1. Gather information.
2. Focus on initial planning components.
3. Examine the training program in more detail.
4. Plan the periodization of each cycle.

Step 1, information gathering, includes determining the athlete's short- and long-term goals, overall focus for the competitive season, and race priorities and objectives. The coach needs to find out about the athlete's current training program and whether the athlete prefers group or individual training. The coach should also identify the current equipment available and any new equipment that will be needed throughout the training program. In addition, the coach should determine what type of terrain (geographical location) is available, as well as the type of environment and climate in that area.

This step also involves determining the athlete's sport background, competitive history, sport-specific strengths and weaknesses, injury history, muscular imbalances, physiological variables (based on lactate threshold, metabolic, and body composition testing), biochemical variables (based on blood work analysis), and biomechanical variables (body movement efficiency patterns). Most important, the coach and the athlete need to determine the amount of time that the athlete can realistically devote to training on a daily basis. This should include identifying the athlete's life commitments (such as family, social, and career) and details on the athlete's daily commute (mode and time to and from work). Many new endurance athletes are a bit overzealous and take on more than they can handle. Athletes must differentiate between realistic and idealistic time goals so that they can achieve a proper balance between sport and life.

Step 2 involves focusing on the initial planning components. These components include the type and frequency of high-quality training sessions, the time between training sessions, the type and frequency of recovery sessions, and the proper build-to-recover ratio of the periodization program (and when this may fluctuate throughout the training year). In this step, the coach and athlete should also determine the mental training and nutritional strategies that will be used. In addition, they should identify the method of communication and type of feedback that will be used between the athlete and coach.

Step 3 begins the process of planning the training program in more detail. This includes determining the specific training techniques that will be used at specific times of the year and throughout the meso- and microcycles. In addition, the coach and athlete should determine when tactical skills will be worked on in relation to race-specific scenarios, determine when and where specific training sessions should be placed throughout each training cycle, and identify the associated goals and outcomes for each specific workout. Athletes need to have specific physical, mental, and nutritional goals for each training session throughout the training plan. Nonquality training sessions are not exempt from this rule. Each training session, regardless of type, should include specific goals and objectives, and recovery opportunities should be emphasized. The structure of recovery sessions throughout the training program should be planned in this step.

The last step includes planning each periodization cycle. In general, the preparatory cycle lasts 12 to 16 weeks. In a traditional periodization plan, the preparatory cycle enables the athlete to build the aerobic foundation, strength, and flexibility needed to progress to the next cycle (the next cycle is more physically, mentally, and nutritionally challenging). The precompetition build cycle is where the goals of improving speed, economy, power, and race-specific strength are normally implemented (in 2- to 8-week cycles). This provides the athlete with optimal recovery time before the race season begins. As the race season approaches, properly implemented tapers will become crucial in getting the athlete to the start line feeling rested and ready to race.

The actual competition season can be quite long—up to 36 weeks for some athletes—but race blocks are often separated into 1- to 4-week periods if competitions will take place each week. This allows the body to recover well. In addition, because most athletes can only achieve two or three formal peaks in the competition season, top-priority competitions are often separated into two or three separate blocks throughout the season. A transition between competitions or intense training blocks can be included in order to implement short recovery bouts between competitions. These recovery bouts usually last 1 or 2 weeks. Additionally, a full transition cycle of 2 to 8 weeks can be scheduled at the end of the competition season. This gives the athlete a full block of recovery. During this transition cycle, the athlete's goals are to exercise without structure, cross-train, have fun, and take a mental and physical reprieve.

Here are some additional things that coaches and athletes need to consider when determining the structure and timing of training cycles:

▶ When and where strength training fits into the program

▶ When to implement drills that require fine movements and a high amount of focus

▶ How many high-quality training sessions should be implemented during each training cycle

▶ Whether two high-quality training sessions should be completed in one day (referred to as combo workouts or bricks for multisport athletes; referred to as doubles for single-sport athletes)

PERIODIZATION

For endurance athletes, the normal progression of fitness begins by developing a good aerobic base (see figure 3.1). Overdistance (OV) and endurance (EN) training are used to build the base of the aerobic system. This is followed by more high-aerobic and tempo work (moving up the pyramid). Then lactate threshold and maximal effort sessions (top of the pyramid) are added when the body has built up a strong foundation of aerobic fitness and strength.

A normal distribution outlining the volume, intensity, and percentage of each type of training during each progression can be seen in table 3.1. As noted, aerobic conditioning (indicated as overdistance and endurance) is a major portion of training year-round. Speed work (indicated as lactate threshold and $\dot{V}O_2max$) is a smaller but very important component of training that helps athletes improve their performance. The information in table 3.1 can be used as a guide for planning the volume, intensity, and relative contributions of each area shown in figure 3.1.

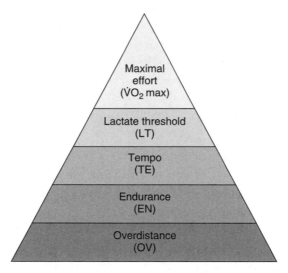

Figure 3.1 Sample traditional periodization progression for endurance athletes.

Two types of periodization are commonly used by endurance athletes: traditional and inverse. Both types can be implemented using a standard or reverse method. In traditional periodization, the athlete progresses through the typical cycles of preparatory (base), precompetition (build or intensity), competition (race), and transition (off-season). For athletes who compete in events, a short tapering phase is generally used before competition. (See Tapering and Peaking later in this chapter.)

Table 3.1   Distribution of Training Load for Each Type of Training

Cycle	Volume	Intensity	Over-distance	Endurance	Tempo	Lactate threshold	V̇O₂max
Preparatory	Moderate to high	Low	60%	30%	5%	5%	0%
Precompetition	Moderate	Moderate to high	55%	25%	5-10%	10-15%	0-10%
Taper	Low to moderate	Moderate to high	55%	25%	5-10%	10-15%	2-5%
Competition	Low to moderate	High	55%	20%	5-10%	5-10%	0-5%
Transition	Low	Low	85%	5-10%	0-5%	0%	0%

Figure 3.2 presents an example of the standard method of building volume and intensity within a traditional plan. The example depicts a 3-week build that should be followed by a 1-week recovery cycle. This strategy is usually best for novice and intermediate endurance athletes who have less than 7 years experience in the sport. The athlete is able to slowly build volume and intensity over 3 weeks. Note that a standard 3:1 build-to-recover progression is merely an example of the many ways to periodize a training program. This method could lead to high fatigue during the third week if the athlete is not ready for the load or if the athlete has a lot of outside stressors that influence recovery.

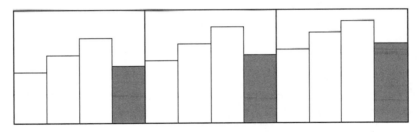

Figure 3.2   Traditional periodization with a standard method of progression.

The reverse method, as its name implies, begins with a higher load and gradually decreases through the cycle (as shown in figure 3.3 on page 50). Athletes who have 7 or more years of experience in the sport can typically handle this type of progression. Because the training load is highest in the first week of training, this strategy is more demanding and should only be used by advanced athletes. This

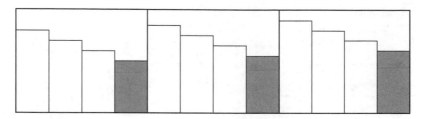

Figure 3.3 Traditional periodization with a reverse method of progression.

method can provide great benefits because the athlete engages in the highest training load after a recovery week, so the body is more rested. The athlete can more easily attain a higher volume and intensity of training because the accumulated fatigue is not as great as it is when using the standard method of progression.

The second popular type of periodization, inverse, begins the training year with an emphasis on strength and technique. The athlete then progresses to focusing on speed and strength, followed by aerobic power and economy. Finally, before the competitive season, the athlete shifts to focusing on aerobic capacity. The two methods of progression—standard and reverse—still apply. Because of the higher speed and the strength training component in the beginning of the training year, athletes should be experienced in their sport and have well-established cardiovascular fitness before beginning this method. This method of progression improves the athlete's strength and speed earlier in the year and allows the aerobic component to be shortened and implemented just before the race season.

As mentioned previously, a periodization mesocycle can be planned in many ways. The traditional 3:1 build-to-recover cycle is popular but is not recommended for all athletes (as explained earlier). Other potential build-to-recover models—such as 2 weeks to 1 week, 16 days to 5 days, or 23 days to 5 days—can be implemented with great success. The 2:1 cycle is especially good for novice endurance athletes because it allows for good recovery in the beginning of a training program. Keep in mind that any single approach to training may not work throughout the entire season. For an athlete to continue progressing toward optimal performance, various training methods may need to be used throughout the athlete's training year. Once the athlete's body begins to develop and the athlete's performance begins to level off, it may be time to change the periodization method or look at the recovery program in more detail.

OVERTRAINING VERSUS OVERLOADING

The term *overtraining* (also known as underrecovery) causes a lot of controversy and confusion. People generally accept that the most important cause of improved performance is the training that athletes undergo, particularly for events that require endurance or superior physical conditioning. Some coaches and athletes believe that there is no limit beyond which training becomes counterproductive. However, there is a limit to an athlete's capacity to withstand and adapt to intense training. Once this threshold is crossed, the athlete fails to adapt, and performance declines.

Overload is a planned, systematic, and progressive increase in training with the goal of improving performance. A zone of positive training adaptation exists where athletes can reap the benefits of their training. However, this has a scale effect; if too little of an acute overload is introduced (known as underreaching), some training adaptations will occur but will only yield small increases in performance. If the athlete maximizes full training adaptations by following a planned overload program that also includes timed recovery periods, performance can increase significantly. Overreaching occurs over the short term when an athlete either has too much training volume or intensity or does not allow adequate recovery. If this situation is not recognized by the athlete or coach, then the short-term overreaching can transition into overtraining. Athletes need to find the balance between underreaching and overreaching, and they should constantly focus on high-quality training sessions within a recovery-based training model. This will yield consistent improvements in performance without the risk of overtraining.

TAPERING AND PEAKING

Competitive athletes perform countless hours of training with the goal of being at the optimal level of performance for the important competitions. As mentioned previously, from a physiological standpoint, an athlete can achieve two or three main peaks in a season. For some athletes, a peak can be maintained for 1 or 2 weeks. This means that they may be able to perform back-to-back races in a peak state. However, the challenge often lies in planning the taper so that the athlete peaks at the right time. Many athletes will miss their peak as a result of an inappropriately timed taper.

A taper can be defined in various ways, but generally speaking, a taper is a progressive reduction in training load. This reduction in the training load is meant to reduce the physical and psychological stressors incurred on a daily basis in order to enhance the body's adaptation to training—and thus optimize performance. Many physical and psychological factors are improved with a properly implemented taper. Two main training variables are usually adjusted for a taper: volume and intensity. Both must be carefully balanced to reap the positive effects.

When a taper is implemented properly, athletes can expect to see a 0.5 to 6.0 percent increase in performance. The most important variable in a taper is intensity. This is often overlooked by athletes and coaches, but intensity needs to be maintained in order to avoid a detraining effect. The frequency of training should be maintained at 80 percent or greater compared to normal; volume should be reduced by 60 to 90 percent over the duration of the taper in order to induce the positive physiological and psychological responses. The duration of the taper requires a bit more planning because the specific requirements will vary by sport and discipline. Research has shown that an optimal taper lasts 4 to 28 days. The specific length of the taper is based on a variety of factors, including athlete experience, length of the event being trained for, and the importance of the competition. Novice athletes or coaches may want to discuss these factors with a more experienced mentor or friend. There is often no rhyme or reason in an athlete's decision on the duration of the taper; however, athletes who compete over shorter distances usually use a shorter taper, and athletes who compete over longer distances usually use a longer taper. Additionally, the type or pattern of the taper will affect whether the athlete can successfully peak and rest. The three patterns of tapers include linear, step, and progressive.

In a linear taper, the volume of training is gradually decreased day by day throughout the duration of the taper (think of walking down stairs). In contrast, a step taper employs a significant reduction (greater than 50 percent) in training volume immediately and then maintains this reduction without fluctuations (think of falling to a lower step all at once and then remaining on that step). The last type, progressive, has been shown to be the most beneficial. In a progressive taper, training is decreased by about 10 to 15 percent immediately, and then gradual decreases are made with a lower-percentage reduction each day (this is a combination of the previous two taper patterns). This pattern allows the necessary reduction in volume to be implemented while maintaining intensity and frequency. Tapering for a race distance can be successful after implementing small "practice" tapers during training. However, tapering becomes more difficult if an athlete competes at different race distances throughout the same year. In this case, the athlete should use a previous successful taper and adjust the taper into smaller increments rather than reinvent the wheel and try something completely different.

Planning an athlete's endurance training program takes knowledge of the various components that make up the program; however, the many variables in the athlete's life and training are also important when fine-tuning the program to meet the athlete's needs. Once the planning stage is complete, the athlete's progress should be continually monitored to assess positive physiological adaptations. Remember, a training program that is effective in bringing about positive physiological adaptations will not necessarily result in optimal adaptations year after year. For the athlete to achieve optimal performance year after year, different goals and strategies must be implemented.

WARM-UP AND COOL-DOWN

Before beginning a workout or race, athletes need to complete a warm-up to prepare the body for activity. The purpose of a warm-up is to increase blood flow to the working muscles and increase core temperature while gradually increasing the intensity of activity. This allows the athlete to be physiologically prepared for the activity to follow. A warm-up typically starts with a general activity and progresses through low-intensity aerobic work that is specific to the workout scheduled. For example, before a running workout, an athlete may begin the warm-up with a slow walk and then gradually increase the exercise intensity. The total time of the warm-up may be as long as 30 minutes. Typically, the higher the intensity of the scheduled activity, the longer the warm-up should be.

The cool-down enables the athlete to progress back to a resting state at the conclusion of activity. This is an important part of the recovery process. The increased blood flow to the working muscles that occurs during activity is slowly redistributed back to the core of the body. The exercise intensity gradually decreases as the cool-down progresses from sport-specific activity to more general movements. This gradual decrease in intensity allows heart rate and body temperature to begin to return to normal. The total time of a cool-down may be as long as 30 minutes. Similar to the warm-up, higher-intensity workouts will require a longer cool-down. Activities that last longer will also require a longer cool-down. This allows the blood in the working muscles to be redistributed back through the body, and it helps the body temperature return to a resting level.

DYNAMIC FLEXIBILITY

Endurance sports are dynamic activities. Muscles contract concentrically and eccentrically, moving the joints of the body through specific motions. Most of the movements used in endurance activities do not require the full range of motion of the joints. Many athletes, especially as they increase their training volumes, find that some joint motions increase while others decrease because of changes in muscle flexibility. Aging has also been linked to decreases in muscle flexibility.

Traditionally, athletes have performed static stretching to improve muscle flexibility. Recent research has suggested that at least some of the work used to increase muscle flexibility should involve dynamic flexibility. Dynamic flexibility exercises are activities that use sport-specific movements to take the joints through a complete range of motion. These sport-specific movements are performed under control and are meant to increase the range of motion of the joints. Before training or competition, a runner who includes dynamic flexibility as part of the warm-up might perform dynamic stretching activities such as walking lunges (for the hip extensors) and walking diagonal lunges (for the abductors).

STATIC STRETCHING

Recently, a growing body of research has reported that static stretching before activity may cause a decrease in power production. This decrease in power production could be important in short-distance, high-intensity endurance events or for athletes striving to maximize performance at a very high level. It could also be detrimental for activities of varying intensities, such as a cycling criterium, which requires intermittent periods of very high-intensity exercise.

Researchers are still exploring the effects of static stretching on performance. However, athletes who want to perform static stretching before activity should also include some general and sport-specific movements. After a workout, static stretching may help relieve muscle soreness, promote relaxation, and increase flexibility. In these instances, static stretching should concentrate on major muscle groups, especially those that are least flexible or those that work in a limited range of motion during training or competition. For example, static stretches for the hip extensors and abductor muscles are a good choice for cyclists and runners because these activities require only limited hip motion.

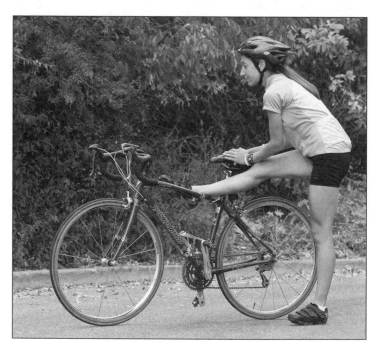

Athletes should use static stretches after exercising to reduce muscle soreness and increase flexibility.

INJURY PREVENTION

Injuries are an inevitable part of endurance training. The optimal race performance or fitness level is achieved by pushing to maximize conditioning without overtraining or injury. A breakthrough performance occurs when the athlete and coach are able to maximize the training load without going too far. Experienced coaches often talk about training their athletes on "the knife edge"—pushing them to maximize adaptations without pushing them over the edge.

Injuries can be placed into two categories: acute and chronic. Acute injuries are those that have an identifiable onset; for example, turning an ankle while running on a trail, or finishing a swim session and noticing shoulder pain. Chronic injuries have a more gradual onset. The athlete may notice pain or discomfort (for part of a workout or after a workout) that subsides after a short period of time. As training progresses, the pain or discomfort may become more severe or may be noticeable for a longer period of time.

The rate and severity of injuries can be reduced by using periodization and by recognizing that stress occurs not just from training and inadequate rest, but also from other areas of life. Poor work conditions, family problems, and trying to do too much all create stress that requires recovery. If athletes try to do too much training, fit too much into their life, or skimp on recovery and rest, they will eventually be unable to recover from the stresses of training. As a result, injuries will occur. Remember, it is better for an athlete to be on the starting line and slightly undertrained than to be overtrained or injured.

If an injury occurs, the athlete needs to be able to identify it before it becomes too severe. Especially at high training volumes, small irritations can become big problems if they are not recognized and dealt with. Athletes must understand the difference between muscle soreness from training and muscle pain from the beginning of an overuse injury. This is something that is difficult to teach, but it is a valuable skill for an athlete to develop.

Athletes can take steps to minimize the loss of training time due to injury. These steps include following a proper training program, allowing adequate recovery from training, and developing a network of medical professionals if injury does occur. A short course of physical therapy, combined with modifications in training, can often reduce the loss of training time from an acute injury—or prevent a slight problem from developing into a chronic injury.

ENVIRONMENTAL CONDITIONS

Environmental conditions can influence the performance of even well-trained and prepared athletes. The environment can dramatically increase the physiological stresses encountered during endurance activity. Extremes in temperature and humidity can result in less-than-optimal performance from even elite athletes. In all environmental conditions, athletes should strive to maintain core temperature, fluid balance, and blood glucose levels while maximizing performance. The combination of exercise stresses and environmental stresses does not allow maintenance of homeostasis, but ideally, the athlete's body can maintain a steady state, or a constant internal environment. Environmental extremes, especially for athletes traveling to unfamiliar environments, make it difficult to maintain a steady state. In response to the heat produced by exercise and the environmental temperature, an athlete's body works to maintain a constant internal environment by attempting to regulate body temperature.

Heat Transfer

The human body is able to gain or lose heat in four ways: conduction, convection, radiation, and evaporation. Conduction is heat transfer from contact between two surfaces. For example, when a person sits on a cold metal bench, heat is conducted from the body to the cooler bench.

Convection is a specific type of conduction that occurs via the transfer of heat between a person and air or fluid. When an athlete is immersed in water (e.g., a triathlete or distance swimmer), the conductive and convective heat exchange that occurs between the athlete and the water is much greater than heat exchange created by other conditions. This is the main reason that wetsuits are allowed for many triathlons. The wetsuit traps a layer of water between the skin and the suit, and it reduces the rate of convective heat loss. Another example of convection in the triathlon occurs during the bike and run. Because of the greater speed of the bike compared to the run, the convective heat exchange is much greater. In fact, during a race, triathletes may not be aware of extreme heat conditions until the start of the run.

Radiation is heat gain or heat loss by way of electromagnetic waves. An extreme example of radiative heat exchange for endurance athletes is the environmental stress seen by Ironman athletes competing on the lava fields of Kona. The athletes absorb heat from the environment, both from the sun and from the heated lava fields.

Evaporation is the conversion of water to water vapor. Athletes lose a lot of heat through the evaporation of sweat. The body loses 580 kilocalories (kcal) of heat for each liter of evaporated sweat. However, if the sweat does not evaporate and soaks clothing or drops to the ground, then no evaporative cooling can occur. The environmental humidity has the greatest effect on the rate of sweat evaporation. The more humid the environment, the lower the level of sweat evaporation. The cooling effect of sweat only occurs when the sweat evaporates. Higher air humidity reduces sweat evaporation.

When exercising in a cold environment, athletes need to be concerned about maintaining core temperature above 95 degrees Fahrenheit in order to avoid developing hypothermia. In cooler environments, heat loss from the body often occurs in windy conditions or when the athlete's clothing becomes wet, such as when a novice competitor wears clothing that does not wick sweat (e.g., a cotton T-shirt). Minimizing skin exposure to the wind and protecting the extremities from the cold can go a long way toward ensuring safe exercise. By taking these precautions, athletes can minimize the occurrence of frostnip (cold damage to the epidermis of the skin) and the more severe frostbite (fluid freezing in and between the skin cells). Many of the effects of cold exposure can be controlled by making well-planned clothing choices. Dressing in layers, using clothing that wicks moisture, and wearing an outer layer that protects against the wind help to minimize the development of cold-related problems.

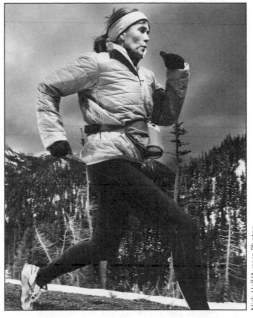

Athletes must wear clothing that helps them maintain proper core temperature in cold and wet conditions.

Open-water swimmers and triathletes need to be aware that heat transfer in the water occurs at least twice as fast as it does on land. This means that these athletes have an increased risk for hypothermia, especially during the longer-distance swims. To help avoid this concern, many triathlons have specific rules that allow wetsuits when water temperatures are below certain levels. However, many open-water swim events do not allow wetsuits. Figure 3.4 on page 58 shows an estimate of survival times with water immersion. The time increases when a wetsuit is worn. Most triathlon swims will not occur in extremely cold water that will be life threatening; however, endurance swimming events in northern parts of the world could take place in temperatures cold enough to be a concern.

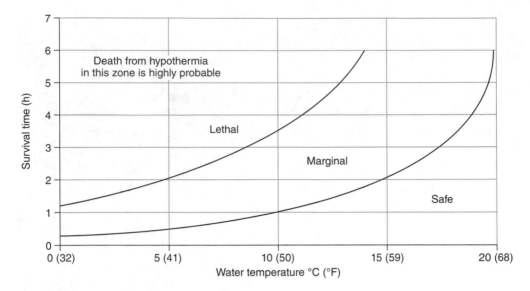

Figure 3.4 Estimated survival time during immersion of lightly clothed, nonexercising humans in cold water. The boundaries (solid lines) would be shifted upward by wearing survival gear or a wet suit.

Adapted, by permission, from L. Armstrong, 2000, *Performing in extreme environments* (Champaign, IL: Human Kinetics), 96. Previously adapted from M.M. Toner and W.D. McArdle, 1998, Physiological adjustments of man to cold. In *Human performance physiology and environmental medicine at terrestrial extremes*, edited by K.B. Pandolf, M.N. Sawka, and R.R. Gonzalez (Indianapolis, Brown & Benchmark), 361-400.

Acclimatization

Proper acclimatization will help an athlete minimize the potential for heat-related problems. A proper acclimatization program will take 10 to 14 days and will involve gradually increasing the exercise intensity and duration. A variety of physiological changes occur during the acclimatization process, including increased sweat rate, increased plasma volume, decreased salt content of the sweat, lower heart rate and core temperature at a given exercise intensity, and increased blood flow to the skin.

An athlete who is unable to be at a race site long enough to acclimate can mimic race conditions by dressing in layers, which acts to create a microenvironment. For a coach who primarily works with athletes in a hot and humid environment, a useful tool to gauge environmental conditions is a sling psychrometer. The psychrometer is used to measure wet bulb global temperature (WBGT). Although coaches and athletes cannot control the environmental conditions, having knowledge of extreme conditions will enable them to modify daily training or race goals. The WBGT is a popular heat stress index. The following equation is used to determine the WBGT:[*]

$$WBGT = (0.7\ T_{wb}) + (0.2\ T_{g}) + (0.1\ T_{db})$$

[*]WBGT equation reprinted from L. E. Armstrong, 2000, *Performing in extreme environments* (Champaign, IL: Human Kinetics), 310.

T_{wb} is the wet bulb temperature, T_g is the black globe temperature, and T_{db} is the shaded dry bulb temperature. The WBGT equation is a more accurate measure of heat stress than ambient temperature. The WBGT takes into account the radiant heat from the sun (T_g) as well as the relationship of environmental humidity (T_{wb}) on heat stress. As you can see from the equation the greatest influence is the humidity (T_{wb}). This is because the main way the body cools itself is via sweat evaporation. The greater the environmental humidity the more difficult it is for sweat to evaporate.

A sling psychrometer typically comes with a chart or table to show the relationship of environmental temperature (T_g), environmental humidity (T_{wb}), and radiant heat (T_{db}) on the risk for heat related problems during exercise.

Heat Illness

Even with acclimatization, athletes and coaches need to be aware of the three forms of heat illness: heat cramps, heat exhaustion, and heatstroke. Heat cramps may affect a single muscle, or in more extreme cases, an athlete may experience whole-body cramping. Athletes who develop heat exhaustion will have a heavy sweat rate, will look pale, and may complain of GI distress or complain of not feeling well in general.

The most serious heat-related problem is heatstroke. The major sign of heatstroke is a lack of sweating (red, hot, and dry skin) in a hot environment. This is a life-threatening condition because sweat evaporation is the major method of heat loss in a hot environment. Keep in mind that heat-related problems—cramps, exhaustion, and stroke—are not sequential; an athlete can develop heatstroke without first having heat cramps or heat exhaustion.

Terrain

Most amateur endurance athletes are not able to travel to a race destination until a few days before the competition. As previously mentioned, this is potentially problematic when athletes need to acclimate to hot and humid environments. Similarly, most athletes do not have the luxury of always training on terrain that is similar to race terrain, especially if the race is held in a hilly or mountainous part of the world. Unfortunately, athletes who live in areas without significant elevation changes will have a difficult time training for the terrain extremes seen at some race venues.

However, with some ingenuity, athletes can create a training situation that partially mimics race conditions. Highway on-ramps, stadium ramps, a bicycle trainer with the front wheel elevated on blocks, and a treadmill with an incline can all help athletes arrive at a race with at least some training that simulates the race terrain.

CHAPTER 4

Endurance Sport Nutrition and Hydration

Bob Seebohar

Most athletes know that improperly fueling or hydrating their body can stop a training session short or lead to the infamous "did not finish" (DNF) during a race. But for various reasons, athletes often fail to give nutrition the same attention that they give to other aspects of training design. Physical periodization—that is, varying the volume and intensity of training throughout the year—is crucial to successful race performance. Altering the daily nutrition plan to support the shifts in training volume and intensity is equally important; this is called nutrition periodization.

This chapter provides a broad overview of nutrition as well as special considerations for effective endurance training. The chapter is designed to provide immediately applicable information for the endurance coach or self-coached athlete. Individuals who want more in-depth information should see the references section of the book on page 285.

NUTRITION PERIODIZATION

Nutrition periodization helps ensure that the athlete receives the nutrients that are needed to enhance health and improve strength, speed, power, and endurance. At the same time, this strategy helps the athlete maintain a healthy immune system and a proper body weight and body composition. Nutrition periodization supports changes in training load so that athletes are able to achieve high-quality workouts and recover more quickly. A nutrition program should vary to meet the athlete's changing energy needs when the athlete trains using a periodized plan. Nutrition supports physical training and enables athletes to train and recover well—and to move toward the goal of improving athletic performance. There is no exception to this, whether an athlete is in the beginning, middle, or end of a training cycle. Nutrition periodization is meant to be a year-long endeavor to support the athlete's changes in energy expenditure.

If an athlete is not nutritionally prepared before a training session, the athlete will not receive the same physiological training adaptations as someone who is prepared and who pays particular attention to nutrition throughout the year. Endurance athletes typically progress through the following training cycles no matter the sport: preparatory (base), precompetition (build or intensity), competition (race), and transition (off-season). Each cycle may last a few weeks or months and may include various physical goals in preparing the athlete for competition. Although sports may blend from season to season, each sport will still progress through a preparatory, competition, and usually an off-season cycle.

The recommended daily macronutrient ranges for endurance athletes (as cited in scientific research) include 3 to 19 grams of carbohydrate per kilogram of body weight, 1.2 to 2.0 grams of protein per kilogram of body weight, and 0.8 to 3.0 grams of fat per kilogram of body weight. (Divide an athlete's body weight in pounds by 2.2 to find the body weight in kilograms.) Keep in mind that these are the ranges reported in the scientific literature. Clearly, the higher values would be extreme, but some of the ultradistance events are also extreme.

MYTH OF THE IDEAL DIET

Athletes often fall into the trap of believing that there is an ideal diet. There is no single diet that is ideal for every athlete. Athletes favor different foods, and the important thing is to ensure that adequate levels of macronutrients (carbohydrate, protein, fat, and water) and micronutrients (vitamins and minerals) are ingested. This can be achieved by eating a variety of foods. Two athletes could eat entirely different foods, but as long as they are achieving adequate macro- and micronutrient intake, they are both consuming an ideal diet.

These recommended daily nutrient ranges are based on information from scientific research that studied various endurance athletes, including cyclists, runners, swimmers, and triathletes. The ranges are large because the research covered athletes ranging from those who compete over very short distances and durations to those who compete in events of very long duration (i.e., athletes who qualify as "ultra" endurance athletes). These ranges will provide a starting point and a foundation of knowledge for people who need to create an eating program to be used in conjunction with a specific training program. The nutrient ranges can be applied directly to endurance athletes in each of the training cycles.

Before using the concept of nutrition periodization, the coach must first have a clear understanding of the physical goals of the athlete. Understanding these goals will help determine which foods should be eaten, the quantity of those foods, and the proper timing of the food intake. Nutrition periodization is designed so that the nutrition needs of an athlete are met. To ensure that the needs are met, the coach must know whether the athlete is attempting to maximize performance, train for health and fitness, or train with the goal of reducing body fat. Once these physical goals are known, the coach can develop the proper nutrition periodization plan.

HYDRATION

Staying hydrated can also have a positive effect on an athlete's performance. In the past, experts provided suggestions on the amount of water all athletes should drink per day. These types of suggestions are no longer made. Hydration is much more individualized; some athletes may require more or less fluid for hydration based on many factors, such as food intake, exercise frequency, exercise intensity, time and type of exercise, sweat rate, and geographical location or environmental conditions.

Without access to the methods used for laboratory analysis, such as using a refractometer to analyze urine specific gravity, athletes can determine their daily hydration needs based on urine color and frequency of urination. After the athlete's first void in the morning (which is not a good measure of hydration), the urine color should be pale yellow to clear and not the color of apple juice. Remember that urine color may not be a good gauge of hydration status for athletes who are taking high levels of some vitamins. Urinating frequently (about every 2 hours) can be a good marker of hydration status. Urine color charts can also be an excellent tool for gauging hydration status.

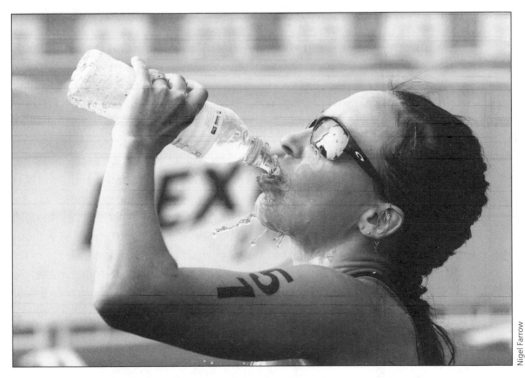

Nigel Farrow

Athletes must maintain fluid balance to avoid the detrimental effects dehydration causes in performance.

COMMON HYDRATION QUESTIONS

Question: Do sports drinks provide benefits that enhance an endurance athlete's body functioning and performance?

Answer: Yes, the palatability or taste of sports drinks increases the likelihood of adequate fluid intake. Carbohydrates and electrolytes are important for optimal metabolic function during exercise.

Question: What are the training and performance consequences of frequent alcohol consumption by an endurance athlete?

Answer: Frequent excessive intake of alcohol will result in the consumption of nutrient-empty calories from the alcohol, dehydration, disrupted sleep patterns, and an increased chance of engaging in risky behaviors.

Question: If the internal "thirst response" isn't a very good gauge, why shouldn't athletes simply drink to the point of not being able to take another sip?

Answer: Although not as common as too little fluid intake, ingesting too much fluid is also possible. Hyponatremia, or water intoxication, occurs when either excessive fluid is ingested or inadequate sodium is consumed to replace what is lost in the sweat. In addition, if an athlete drinks at a rate faster than fluid can be absorbed (about 1 liter per hour for most individuals), then the fluid will stay in the gut, increasing the risk of gastric distress.

Keep in mind that water is not the only way to meet daily fluid requirements. Because of personal preference, many athletes will not drink plain water. For these athletes, eating foods that have a high water content, such as fruits and vegetables, can help them stay hydrated. Significant dehydration can be detrimental to performance; thus, athletes should always strive to stay in fluid balance, whether from drinking plain water or eating foods with a high water content.

Another important aspect of hydration is electrolyte balance. Electrolytes are substances that are able to conduct electricity. In the human body, sodium (Na), chloride (Cl), potassium (K), and calcium (Ca) are the four electrolytes that are considered the most important. These electrolytes help conduct neural signals, maintain proper fluid levels in cells, and maintain proper concentrations of various body fluids (blood, cerebral spinal fluid, and so on). During exercise, electrolytes are lost through sweat; small amounts are also lost through the urine. This is one of the reasons why sports drinks contain small levels of these electrolytes—to allow replenishment of those lost during exercise.

FEMALE ATHLETE TRIAD

The female athlete triad is a combination of three interrelated conditions: energy deficit (disordered eating), menstrual disturbances (amenorrhea), and bone loss (osteoporosis). The triad is most common in females participating in sports that promote a lean physique (gymnastics, figure skating, cross country running, ballet, swimming, diving) or sports that require weight checks. It is also common in female athletes who have controlling parents or coaches. The three conditions that make up the female athlete triad are interrelated because of their effects on each other. Energy deficiency plays a role in the development of menstrual disturbances; energy deficiency (along with low estrogen) also plays a role in initiating bone loss.

One of the primary causes of the triad is chronic energy deficiency. In some cases, the amount of food that athletes eat is not enough to meet their energy expenditure. The energy deficiency can be caused by consuming too few calories to support training or by burning too many calories through training without adequate replacement of food calories. Some form of disordered eating behavior is usually associated with the energy deficiency. This is driven by the athlete's desire to be thin or to achieve a low body weight. Some of the common signs and symptoms of the triad include the following:

- Sleep problems
- Constant fatigue and tiredness
- Irregular or absent menstrual cycles
- Stress fractures
- Striving to be thin
- Restriction of food
- Cold hands and feet

Most of the efforts to educate female athletes about the triad have focused on nutrition and disordered eating. The best strategies for helping athletes who show signs of the female athlete triad include reminding the athletes that eating is just as important as training and that food plays a crucial role in performance and recovery. These strategies also include focusing on health and a positive body image and using a team of professionals, including sport dietitians, physicians, counselors, and certified athletic trainers.

YEAR-ROUND NUTRITION PROGRAM

By implementing a year-round nutrition program in conjunction with their training program, endurance athletes can reap the benefits of enhanced health, improved performance, and better control of weight and body composition. Remember that the eating program should ebb and flow just as the training does; the athlete's physical performance will be much more supported when nutrition matches the needs of physical training. The most important nutrients to consume during training are carbohydrate, fluid, and electrolytes. Table 4.1 provides recommendations for the intake of carbohydrate, protein, and fat during each training cycle. These recommendations are discussed in further detail in upcoming sections.

Table 4.1 Nutrition Periodization Nutrient Ranges by Training Cycle

Training cycle	Carbohydrate	Protein	Fat
Preparatory (no weight loss goals)	4-7 g/kg	1.2-1.7 g/kg	0.8-1.0 g/kg
Preparatory (with weight loss goals)	3-4 g/kg	1.8-2.0 g/kg	0.8 g/kg
Competition	7-15 g/kg	1.4-1.6 g/kg	0.8-1.5 g/kg
Transition	3-4 g/kg	1.6-2.0 g/kg	0.8-1.0 g/kg

Reprinted, by permission, from B. Seebohar, 2011, *Nutrition periodization for athletes: Taking traditional sports nutrition to the next level*, 2nd ed. (Boulder, CO: Bull Publishing).

COMMON ERRORS IN NUTRITION PROGRAMS

Endurance athletes commonly make the following two errors in carrying out their nutrition programs:

- **Inadequate hydration during and after training.** Hydration is essential for optimal performance and optimal recovery. Athletes who ingest too little fluid will compromise the effectiveness of training and will increase the length of time it takes to recover from training.

- **Not maintaining an appropriate nutrient intake on a day-to-day basis.** Athletes and coaches need to recognize that ingesting too many calories is just as detrimental as ingesting too few calories. Ingesting too many calories can lead to weight gain, usually in the form of adipose. Ingesting too few calories minimizes training effectiveness and the recovery from training. Nutrition periodization helps ensure that nutrient intake is based on training load.

Nutrition for the Preparatory Cycle

In addition to the athlete's physical goals, losing weight and improving body composition may also be a high priority during the preparatory cycle. Daily carbohydrate intake depends on body weight and activity level:

▶ For moderate-duration and low-intensity training (1 to 3 hours per day), the recommended daily intake is 4 to 7 grams per kilogram of body weight.

▶ For moderate to heavy training (3 to 4 hours per day), the recommended daily intake is 7 to 10 grams per kilogram of body weight.

▶ For extreme training (4 to 6 hours or more per day), the recommended daily intake is 10 or more grams per kilogram of body weight.

Most endurance athletes will not likely fall into the extreme training category during this cycle. Until training volume significantly increases, a general recommendation is that the majority of carbohydrates come from fruits and vegetables, because these foods contain a good balance of beneficial vitamins, minerals, antioxidants, and fiber. A good goal would be to eat 6 to 12 servings of fruits and vegetables per day. This may sound like a lot, but the serving sizes of fruits and vegetables are fairly small. Athletes can distribute the servings throughout the day by eating 1 or 2 servings every meal and snack. This makes it much easier to ensure that an adequate amount is eaten. Whole grains can be included in controlled amounts to satisfy carbohydrate needs.

Daily protein intake can range from 1.2 to 1.7 grams per kilogram of body weight depending on the athlete's goals for body weight. Athletes should choose the leanest sources of protein, such as low-fat dairy products and lean cuts of meat, chicken, turkey, or fish without skin or visible fat.

The recommended amount of fat to be consumed on a daily basis remains relatively low at 0.8 to 1.0 grams per kilogram of body weight. The types of fat that are most beneficial include monounsaturated (found in avocados, olives, and nuts) and polyunsaturated, specifically omega-3 fats (found in salmon, trout, walnuts, and flax products). At all costs, athletes need to minimize the intake of saturated and trans fats found in processed and snack foods and high-fat meats.

Some athletes make losing weight and reducing body composition a primary goal during the preparatory training cycle. If an athlete falls into this category, the recommended daily intake of carbohydrate should be reduced to 3 or 4 grams per kilogram of body weight. A higher amount of protein—from 1.8 to 2.0 grams per kilogram of body weight per day—should be included; this intake of protein should have a special emphasis on branched-chain amino acids because they have a higher satiety factor (they keep a person fuller), which will help stabilize blood sugar. A person with a stable blood sugar level will eat less throughout the day, so including a good source of lean protein at each meal and snack is important. Continue to keep fat intake around 0.8 grams per kilogram of body weight.

Fueling for Training Sessions During the Preparatory Cycle

Staying hydrated and maintaining carbohydrate stores are key components when it comes to eating during any training session. However, the nutrition recommendations are highly variable based on environmental conditions, weight goals, sweat rate, and training load. These variables change as the athlete progresses through the preparatory training cycle. The athlete's nutrition plan should adapt accordingly; however, the following recommendations provide a starting point.

Staying hydrated is the most important factor during the sessions in this cycle. The most recent general guidelines on hydration recommend the following:

drinking 0.07 to 0.10 ounce (2.1-3 ml) of fluid per pound (0.45 kg) of body weight 4 hours before training and an additional 0.04 to 0.10 ounce (1.2-3 ml) of fluid per pound of body weight 2 hours before training if the athlete's urine is not pale yellow in color. For example, a 150-pound (68 kg) athlete would drink 10.5 to 15 ounces (~310-444 ml) of fluid 4 hours before training and an additional 6 to 15 ounces (177-444 ml) of fluid 2 hours before a training session. For endurance athletes who train early in the morning, this is not realistic; thus, the recommendation for these athletes is that they consume at least 0.04 ounce (1.2 ml) of fluid per pound of body weight in the 30 to 45 minutes before training.

If losing weight or body fat is not a goal for the preparatory cycle, athletes should consume 30 to 50 grams of carbohydrate per hour of training. Current recommendations for carbohydrate intake during preparatory cycle training are based on absolute values rather than relative values (grams per kilogram of body weight). The training sessions in this cycle are usually low to moderate volume and low intensity, so athletes do not need more carbohydrate than the basic recommendation. Additional carbohydrate is needed only when the volume and intensity increase during later training cycles.

Athletes can consume carbohydrate from a variety of sources, including solids (crackers, bananas, energy bars) and liquids (sports drinks, gels). Keep in mind that during low- to moderate-intensity exercise, blood flow to the stomach is adequate, which means most athletes should be able to choose easily digestible carbohydrate (i.e., those that have less fiber and are more simple in nature). However, during higher-intensity exercise, blood flow to the stomach is lower, which means solid forms of carbohydrate will probably be more difficult to digest. Protein is typically not needed in high amounts, if at all, during most training sessions in the preparatory cycle.

As mentioned earlier, many individual aspects of hydration must be considered, but in general, athletes should drink 3 to 8 ounces (89-237 ml) of fluid every 15 to 20 minutes during exercise in order to remain hydrated. Of course, this will depend greatly on the training environment, because sweat rates can be drastically different from a hot and humid climate to a cold and dry climate. Cyclists can usually absorb fluid at a greater rate than weight-bearing athletes such as runners. This is partially because cycling uses a smaller muscle mass, which allows more blood flow to the gut and thus helps with gastric emptying. Triathletes must find that delicate balance between drinking enough to maintain hydration status but not drinking so much that it has a negative effect during the run portion of training or racing.

Athletes who are actively trying to lose weight should consider a sports drink that contains electrolytes only; these sports drinks are useful in this situation, especially for low-intensity training sessions shorter than 90 minutes. The individual training sessions within each training cycle will dictate hydration somewhat.

That is the point in using nutrition periodization. The body has enough glycogen to fuel moderate-intensity exercise. If an athlete seeks weight loss and eats before the training session, then extra calories are not needed during this training cycle. Consuming extra calories will slow the progress of weight loss.

After training, the athlete needs to replace the nutrients that were lost. Four nutrients—fluid, carbohydrate, protein, and sodium—are the main focal points for postworkout nutrition and should be consumed immediately after and up to 60 minutes after a session is finished. In the case of fluids, athletes may need to consume quantities greater than those lost. This will help ensure that the necessary fluid levels are adequately restored before the next training session. Drinking 150 percent of fluid losses will help the body rehydrate. Drinking 24 ounces (710) of fluid for every pound (0.45 kg) of body weight lost during the training session is a good practice to follow. Including at least 500 milligrams of sodium in the fluid consumed after exercise will help the body retain the fluid consumed.

If the training session taxed glycogen stores by lasting longer than 90 minutes or by including very high-intensity intervals, postworkout recovery can be enhanced by consuming carbohydrate sources with a higher glycemic index. The athlete should consume 1.0 to 1.2 grams of these sources per kilogram of body weight. High-glycemic carbohydrates include food sources containing high levels of sugar and sources that are highly processed (e.g., most sports drinks). Consuming this type of postworkout snack is easy to do by choosing low-fat chocolate milk, a lean-meat bagel sandwich, or a milk-based fruit smoothie.

Postworkout protein is needed for optimal recovery, although not at the same levels as carbohydrate. Protein intake helps the body shift into positive protein balance. Athletes should eat 10 to 20 grams of high-quality protein (composed mostly of essential amino acids). The postworkout snacks listed previously also meet the postworkout protein requirements needed for optimal recovery. Fat is typically not needed in the "window of opportunity" after a training session and should not be included immediately after exercise.

After the initial postworkout nutrition protocol, athletes who are not seeking weight loss should eat another 1.0 to 1.2 grams of carbohydrate per kilogram of body weight 2 hours after the initial carbohydrate intake; they should repeat this in 2-hour increments throughout the next 6 to 8 hours. This strategy will refill glycogen stores the fastest, typically within 12 to 16 hours instead of 24 hours. (Athletes who are actively trying to lose weight should not follow this regimen; after a moderate training session, these athletes should simply have a small snack of carbohydrate, protein, a little sodium, and some water.)

During this time, any combination of carbohydrates is beneficial as long as they are less processed and refined. Ideas include carbohydrate-rich snacks or meals balanced with lean protein such as a lean turkey sandwich with tomato, lettuce, cucumbers, pickles, and mustard; a nonfat milk or yogurt-based fruit smoothie; a bowl of whole-grain cereal with berries and skim milk; or oatmeal made with skim milk and raisins or other dried fruit. The goal is to maximize glycogen repletion; therefore, smaller snacks or meals are preferred over larger meals that fill the athlete up so much that she cannot eat again in another 2 hours.

Nutrition for the Competition Cycle

For endurance athletes, the competition cycle usually includes the build (pre-competition) and race (competition) components. The build component is often high-intensity and high-volume work aimed at improving speed, power, and sport-specific strength. This adds stress to the body, and recovery is crucial to the athlete's ability to achieve optimal performance. During the competition cycle, the training intensity and volume are also typically quite high. Therefore, athletes should not pursue active weight loss during this cycle.

Some athletes may want to restrict calories in this cycle to try to lose those last few pounds; however, this can be detrimental to higher-intensity training. Caloric restriction prevents the body from maintaining high levels of output and from recovering quickly after intense training sessions. The biggest mistakes made during this time of the season are not eating frequently enough, making poor food choices, and having inadequate fluid intake. The worst thing an athlete can do during the competition season is to significantly alter the nutrition plan.

Because of the higher intensity and frequency of glycogen-depleting workouts, daily carbohydrate intake should increase from the previous training cycle and should range from 7 to 10 grams per kilogram of body weight. For athletes engaging in extreme training, daily carbohydrate intake may need to be greater than 10 grams per kilogram of body weight in order to meet glycogen resynthesis needs. This is not the time for athletes to deny their body the necessary carbohydrate that will be crucial in attaining their workout and recovery goals.

The recommended range for daily intake of protein remains moderate at 1.2 to 1.7 grams per kilogram of body weight. Athletes can use the higher end of this range if their training requires frequent, intense speed training sessions and strength training sessions. The range for fat is similar to the range during the preparatory cycle with the exception of athletes training for ultradistance races; for these athletes, daily fat intake may be as high as 1.5 grams per kilogram of body weight. The higher fat intake for these athletes is needed because of the higher levels of energy loss from longer-duration training sessions. Fat is more energy dense and will help these athletes remain in energy balance. The athletes should focus on healthier fats such as polyunsaturated (specifically omega-3) and monounsaturated fats. They should consume minimal amounts of saturated and trans fat.

Regardless of the training cycle, recommendations for hydration are fairly consistent. Remember, though, that environmental conditions and travel must be taken into account, because these factors can make it more difficult for athletes to stay hydrated.

Fueling for Training Sessions During the Competition Cycle

For training sessions during the competitive cycle, proper fueling allows athletes to achieve optimal effectiveness in the workout and ensures adequate nutrient intake for the recovery process. The nutrient intake before a training session is designed to ensure that the athlete begins the session properly hydrated and with normal levels of muscle glycogen. During the session, the goal is to maintain fluid, electrolyte, and blood glucose levels. Nutrients consumed after the training session allow the athlete to replace fluid, electrolyte, and muscle glycogen stores. Postworkout nutrients also aid the body in recovery from the stress of the training session.

In this cycle, athletes need to prevent or minimize gastrointestinal (GI) distress during training and racing. In the previous discussion on fueling for training during the preparatory cycle, some recommendations were provided for avoiding GI distress, including not consuming high-fiber or high-protein foods and not drinking too much water. These recommendations also apply in the competitive phase. Athletes should rely on their experience during training sessions in the previous cycles to learn how their gut responds to various types and quantities of foods and sport nutrition products. These experiences should be carried over into this training cycle with the intent of topping off fluid, electrolyte, and carbohydrate stores before training.

Newer research has shown that consuming a large amount (144 grams) of carbohydrate per hour during exercise increases the body's ability to oxidize (use) this fuel for energy, thus allowing the body to have a greater fuel supply.

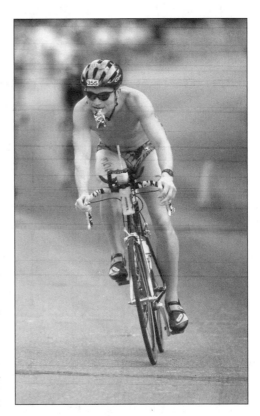

Athletes should consume carbohydrate while training and racing to maintain their fuel supplies.

However, because of the very large carbohydrate intake needed to see these types of oxidation rates, some athletes may find that ingesting this much carbohydrate is simply not realistic. The fact that all of this research was conducted on cyclists should also be taken into consideration. Cyclists may be able to ingest a higher level of nutrition during exercise compared to other forms of exercise that require the use of larger amounts of muscle mass and that are weight bearing activities.

Based on current research, the recommendation for athletes in the competition cycle is to consume from 30 to 90 total grams of carbohydrate per hour during training sessions and competitions. Smaller athletes, especially females, should choose the lower quantities. Larger athletes may be able to consume amounts on the higher end, but they should do so in a race only after trying it with success during training sessions that simulate race intensity. As noted previously, the way that the body digests food at higher intensities can be very different from the way it does at lower intensities.

After a glycogen-depleting workout, athletes should follow the same nutrition guidelines described for the preparatory cycle. They should put special emphasis on consistency. Athletes need to treat their postworkout nutrition regimen as a part of their training session; they must be sure not to forget or delay this regimen.

Nutrition for the Transition or Off-Season Cycle

Most athletes welcome the off-season as a time of rest, recovery, and rejuvenation. However, this is also a time when many athletes make nutritional mistakes and gain unnecessary body fat. These mistakes can occur if an athlete does not continue to emphasize controlled intake of high-quality food. During the off-season cycle, the primary nutrition goal should be to control the amount of food eaten. Controlling blood sugar by eating lean protein and fiber-rich food (fruits and vegetables are preferred) is the main objective.

Additionally, most athletes do not follow a specific training plan during this cycle, even though they may think they do. Rather, they participate in unstructured exercise. Because of the unstructured training, products such as energy bars, gels, sports drinks, and powders are typically not necessary. Because of the lower energy requirements, the recommended daily intake of carbohydrate decreases to as low as 3 or 4 grams per kilogram of body weight; the emphasis should be mostly on fruits and vegetables and less on whole grains and healthier starches. Daily protein intake should range from 1.6 to 2.0 grams per kilogram of body weight. Daily fat intake should remain low at 0.8 to 1.0 grams per kilogram of body weight; the emphasis should be on omega-3 fats.

Fueling for Exercise Sessions
During the Transition or Off-Season Cycle

During this cycle, energy expenditure during training will be lower because training intensity and volume are low. The athlete usually doesn't have specific goals for training improvement. The athlete should focus on being nourished and hydrated before exercise by eating a light, balanced meal or snack. During exercise, the athlete will probably not need more than 8 ounces (~237 ml) of water every 20 to 30 minutes. If needed, small amounts of sodium may be added to the water (500 milligrams of sodium per liter of water) to help the athlete maintain hydration status.

For postexercise nutrition, the athlete should simply focus on replenishing hydration stores by drinking 24 ounces (710 ml) of water (with at least 500 milligrams of sodium per liter of water) immediately after the workout. To enhance postworkout recovery, the athlete can eat a light snack or meal that is low in fat and includes a good source of carbohydrate and some lean protein.

ERGOGENIC AIDS

Among athletes, a lot of confusion exists about ergogenic aids. This confusion is often related to safety and efficacy concerns. Because ergogenic aids are not included in the category of macro- or micronutrients, people often think of them only as performance enhancing and for specific use in sport. Although studies have provided good data to support the performance- and recovery-enhancing effects of some ergogenic aids, a comprehensive review of the most popular supplements is beyond the scope of this chapter.

Excellent texts devoted to the topic of ergogenic aids are available, including *Power Eating, Third Edition* (2007) by Susan Kleiner with Maggie Greenwood-Robinson or *Advanced Sports Nutrition, Second Edition* (2012) by Dan Benardot (both published by Human Kinetics). Coaches and athletes interested in learning more about potential ergogenic aids should seek out these texts. However, athletes should use ergogenic aids under the close supervision of a qualified health professional and should make sure they have a clear understanding of the potential risks.

CHAPTER 5

Aerobic Endurance Development

Will Kirousis
Jason Gootman

Endurance sports typically require participants to traverse extended distances as rapidly as possible. These sports include running, cycling, swimming, triathlon, ultradistance events, and others. Sustaining a good pace in an endurance event and improving that pace require effective, dedicated training. This chapter explains how endurance athletes can properly stress their body during workouts, describes how athletes should treat their body between training sessions, and introduces key factors for achieving optimal stamina in a sport.

TYPES OF WORKOUTS

The cultures of most endurance sports have deep traditions of focusing on completing as many miles and hours as possible, regardless of the quality of the workouts—and even at the expense of quality. This leads to a real challenge for modern-day endurance athletes. With the many outside demands on athletes' time and energy, athletes need time-efficient ways to train effectively that allow them to recover from their workouts and grow stronger. High-quality workouts enable athletes to get the most from the time and energy put into workouts. The benefit of high-quality workouts far exceeds the benefit of completing as many workouts as possible. Athletes should eliminate workouts that do not focus on quality.

In addition to the "more is better" mind-set in society and in the cultural histories of endurance sports, athletes may also feel bombarded with a sea of information on training methods that have accompanied developments in technology. Multitudes of complex training approaches are now available as well as high-tech gadgets and software to dissect and analyze (and overanalyze) training. But at the end of the day, developing endurance still comes down to doing workouts that apply stresses that challenge athletes to cover ground for extended distances as rapidly as they can.

Athletes should focus on simple workouts with clear objectives. Doing so frees athletes to work hard and enjoy their sport. This is the most direct path to success and excellence. To achieve that success and excellence, athletes should use three main endurance-building tools:

▶ **Long workouts.** These workouts are the most specific, and as the training year advances, the workouts can progress to distances similar to an athlete's peak races; in addition, significant portions of the workouts are completed at race intensity. Athletes cannot do in a race what they have not done in a workout (with a few exceptions), and long workouts prepare athletes most specifically for peak races. Not only do these workouts develop the exact physical abilities that are needed for racing, but they also aid tremendously in developing optimal mental abilities. Long workouts are also the ideal chance to practice and experiment with race nutrition and equipment outside of a race.

▶ **Interval workouts.** These high-work and moderate-duration workouts (also known as anaerobic workouts and anaerobic endurance workouts) last less than 1 hour and 30 minutes, which is typically the amount of time that an endurance athlete has available for working out on most days of the week. Interval workouts are potentially the most potent, but they also present the most stress on an athlete. As discussed in chapter 3, athletes should use a planned, systematic, and progressive overload in order to avoid overtraining (sometimes referred to as underrecovery syndrome). Many experienced endurance coaches and athletes will tell you that being slightly undertrained on race day is better than being overtrained.

▶ **Aerobic workouts.** These moderate-work and moderate-duration workouts (also known as aerobic workouts or aerobic endurance workouts) are conservative sessions designed to enhance endurance. Aerobic workouts include a cap or ceiling on intensity that keeps the work almost exclusively aerobic in nature. As a result, these workouts are less effective at developing endurance than interval workouts, but they are also easier to recover from. Blending the right amount of these two types of workouts (used along with long workouts) is part of the art of training.

Interval workouts are made up of higher-intensity work broken up by rest intervals. Both interval workouts (high work, moderate duration) and aerobic workouts (moderate work, moderate duration) can be done as intervals or as steady, uninterrupted periods of work. However, the term *interval workouts* is more commonly used for anaerobic workouts. That's why the terms *intervals* and *interval workouts* are typically used synonymously with *high-work workouts,* and the term *aerobic workouts* is typically used synonymously with *moderate-work workouts.*

Various subclasses of workouts can be categorized within the three types of endurance workouts. This is particularly true of interval workouts, which include hill workouts (cycling and running), fartlek workouts, and interval workouts done on an indoor trainer (cycling), track (running), or treadmill (running).

LONG WORKOUTS

Long workouts are the most specific workouts that athletes can do. These workouts are also the best preparation for races. Because long workouts take up the most time and energy, athletes will typically do only one to three long workouts per week. Triathletes should do one for each discipline. Runners should generally do one long run each week. Cyclists and mountain bike racers can do two long workouts each week, one that is a competitive group ride and one that is a long ride done entirely at aerobic intensity.

The key to effective long workouts is that they challenge athletes to (1) learn to go longer and (2) learn to move at the intensity they will use in their peak races. Simply training without specific goals is not a productive use of time for a competitive athlete. Athletes will get much more out of long workouts that challenge them to move at intensities similar to those used in their peak races. It is unrealistic to expect an athlete to perform long runs at 9 minutes per mile and then race a marathon at 7 minutes per mile. Consider long workouts that include portions at race intensity to be the perfect "tempo workouts" or "pace workouts" to use with athletes. These workouts challenge the athletes to train at an intensity similar to that required for a race.

Athletes should be well rested when they begin a long workout. Therefore, easier workouts or a rest day should be scheduled for the day before a long workout. Long workouts should be completed on a course and in conditions similar to those for the athlete's race. These workouts serve as practice races, so they provide the perfect opportunity to practice with race equipment.

Consider a triathlete training for a half Ironman. Long swims are the perfect chance to practice swimming a distance similar to the race distance—and at race intensity—in a wetsuit. This allows the athlete to get comfortable with the wetsuit, work out any kinks that may exist in the fit of the wetsuit, try a few different wetsuits if necessary, and practice swimming in the wetsuit as he will in races. Bricks (bike-run combination workouts) are a good chance to try out a new cycling position and experiment with equipment in general. The best strategy is usually to test things out in shorter workouts first, then in long workouts.

The distance for long workouts should progress as the training year progresses. Table 5.1 presents a sample long-run progression for a half marathon runner. This table shows long workouts for the 11 weeks before the athlete's taper phase for her peak race.

Each long run is composed of portions to be run at aerobic intensity and portions to be run at race intensity. In week 7 of the progression, for example, the runner would perform a 10-mile (16 km) run. The first 5 miles (8 km) are at aerobic intensity, and the last 5 miles are at race intensity. Athletes should always do the aerobic miles first and the race miles last. This is especially important for running. If an athlete performs the race miles first, fatigue may prevent the athlete from completing the workout or may cause a change in running form that could lead to injury. This concept is less of a consideration in non-weight-bearing activities such as cycling or swimming. The runs should increase in difficulty in two ways as they progress: (1) They get longer, and (2) they involve more miles being run at race intensity. Both factors increase gradually to allow the runner to adapt and get

Table 5.1 Sample Progression of Long Runs for a Half Marathon Runner

Week	Total distance in miles (km)	Distance in miles at aerobic intensity (km)	Distance in miles at race intensity (km)
1	7 (11.2)	6 (9.7)	1 (1.6)
2	7 (11.2)	5 (8)	2 (3.2)
3	9 (14.4)	7 (11.2)	2 (3.2)
4	–	–	–
5	8 (12.9)	3 (4.8)	5 (8)
6	9 (14.4)	5 (8)	4 (6.4)
7	10 (16)	5 (8)	5 (8)
8	–	–	–
9	11 (17.7)	7 (11.2)	5 (8)
10	13 (20.9)	5 (8)	8 (12.9)
11	13 (20.9)	3 (4.8)	10 (16)

Table 5.2 Sample Progression of Brick Workouts for an Ironman Triathlete

Week	Total cycling miles (km)	Cycling miles at aerobic intensity (km)	Cycling miles at race intensity (km)	Running miles at race intensity (km)
1	60 (96.5)	30 (48.2)	30 (48.2)	3 (4.8)
2	75 (121)	30 (48.2)	45 (72)	4 (6.4)
3	100 (160)	30 (48.2)	70 (112.6)	5 (8)
4	–	–	–	–
5	75 (121)	20 (32)	55 (88.5)	6 (9.7)
6	100 (160)	20 (32)	80 (128.7)	8 (12.9)
7	75 (121)	20 (32)	55 (88.5)	6 (9.7)
8	–	–	–	–
9	80 (128.7)	15 (24.1)	65 (105)	8 (12.9)
10	90 (144.8)	15 (24.1)	75 (121)	8 (12.9)
11	100 (160)	15 (24.1)	85 (136.7)	8 (12.9)

better at running longer distances at race intensity. In the example, weeks 4 and 8 are rest weeks, so the athlete does not perform any long runs. After week 11, the runner would have a taper phase of 2 to 3 weeks leading into her race.

As another example, table 5.2 shows a sample progression of bricks for an Ironman triathlete. Again, the total length of the workouts increases as well as the portion performed at race intensity.

Long Run (10K Runner)

The athlete runs 10 total miles (16 km). The first 4 miles (6.4 km) should be run at aerobic intensity. The last 6 miles (9.7 km) are run at race intensity. After completing the run, the athlete should walk for 10 minutes to cool down.

Long Run (Marathon Runner)

The athlete runs 18 total miles (29 km). He runs the first 10 miles at aerobic intensity and the last 8 miles (12.9 km) at race intensity. Then, the athlete should walk for 10 minutes to cool down.

Long Run (Half-Ironman Triathlete)

The athlete runs 12 total miles (19.3 km). The first 6 miles are run at aerobic intensity, and the last 6 miles (9.7 km) are run at race intensity. Then the athlete walks for 10 minutes to cool down.

Long Run (Ironman Triathlete)

The athlete runs 16 total miles (25.7 km). The first 10 miles should be run at aerobic intensity, and the last 6 miles (9.7 km) are completed at race intensity. After completing the run, the athlete walks for 10 minutes to cool down.

Brick (Olympic-Distance Triathlete)

The athlete rides 35 miles total (56.3 km). She rides the first 15 miles (24.1 km) at aerobic intensity and the last 20 miles (32.2 km) at race intensity. After the ride, the athlete runs 4 miles (6.4 km) at race intensity. After completing the run, the athlete walks for 10 minutes to cool down.

Brick (Ironman Triathlete)

The athlete rides 90 miles (144.8 km) total. He rides the first 50 miles (80.5 km) at aerobic intensity and then rides the last 40 miles (64.4 km) at race intensity. After the ride, the athlete runs 4 miles (6.4 km) at race intensity. After completing the run, the athlete walks for 10 minutes to cool down.

Group Ride (Cyclist)

The athlete completes a competitive group ride with other cyclists over a 65-mile (105 km) course. During the ride, the athletes should use competitive tactics commonly used in cycling races. After completing the ride, the athlete rides for 10 minutes at a very low intensity to cool down.

Long Ride (Cyclist)

The athlete rides 75 miles (121 km) at aerobic intensity. After completing the ride, the athlete rides for 10 minutes at a very low intensity to cool down.

INTERVAL WORKOUTS

High-work, moderate-duration workouts are effective for improving endurance. These workouts last from 45 minutes to 1 hour and 30 minutes. The focus is a set of intervals in which the work intervals are completed at anaerobic intensity and the rest intervals are completed at an easy intensity. The following is a good structure for interval workouts:

1. **Warm-up or drill sets.** The purpose of a warm-up is to prepare the body for the higher-intensity work done in the actual workout. The activity starts at a low intensity and increases gradually to allow physiological preparation for the workout. Increased blood flow to the working muscles will occur as the heart rate increases. The increased blood flow will allow the muscle temperature to increase, which in turn will improve the metabolic function of the muscle. Drill sets are an excellent warm-up activity. The drill sets enable the athlete to work on improving specific skills or techniques necessary for the sport. The sport-specific chapters on running, swimming, and biking all have suggested drills to include in training. These drills can also be incorporated into a triathlete's workouts for the individual sports.

2. **Sprint set (optional).** Sprint sets are typically used only by experienced athletes who are working to maximize their performance. The purpose of sprint sets is to improve neuromuscular function, or in simple terms, to teach the athlete what it feels like to move very quickly. Sprint sets generally consist of very short intervals done at an extremely high intensity. The athlete should be encouraged to try to perform the sets without "trying too hard." The idea is to get the athlete familiar with moving at a high rate of velocity without the set causing excessive fatigue. The sets will be mentally fatiguing because of the concentration required, but the athlete should not work so hard that the sprint set causes a high level of physical fatigue.

3. **Main sets (endurance sets).** Generally speaking, for cycling and running, the main sets should consist of 20 to 40 minutes of work intervals done at anaerobic intensity and separated by rest intervals. For swimming, 1,000 to 2,000 yards (914 to 1,829 m) is a good distance for the main sets for most athletes.

4. **Cool-down.** The purpose of a cool-down is the opposite of a warm-up. A cool-down works to decrease blood flow to the working muscles, slow metabolic processes, and allow the body to gradually return to a resting state. Low-intensity activity is commonly used to help with the redistribution of blood and the removal of metabolites from the muscles. This activity allows the athlete to begin recovering from the training session.

As explained in chapter 2, one way that work intensity is measured is with intensity levels. The four levels are easy intensity, aerobic intensity, anaerobic intensity, and race intensity. This method of measuring intensity is easy to use and does not require athletes to use any specialized equipment. The following are some sample workouts that show how these intensity levels are used.

Cycling Hill Workout (Cyclist or Triathlete)

While riding to a hill, the athlete builds in intensity from easy to aerobic as a warm-up (approximately 15 minutes). At the hill, the athlete performs a set of 10 × 3 minutes, riding at anaerobic intensity up the hill; the athlete uses a cadence of 55 to 70 revolutions per minute (rpm). The rest interval is the coast down the hill (the athlete practices descending). After completing the workout, the athlete cools down by riding home, descending in intensity from aerobic to easy (approximately 15 minutes).

Cycling Indoor Trainer Workout (Cyclist or Triathlete)

The athlete begins the workout by riding for 5 minutes to warm up, building in intensity from easy to aerobic. The athlete then performs a set of drills, followed by a sprint set (optional). Next, the athlete performs a set of 15 × 2 minutes, riding at anaerobic intensity; the athlete uses a cadence of 85 to 95 rpm. Between each 2-minute interval, the athlete should rest by riding at easy intensity for 1 minute. To cool down after the workout, the athlete rides for 10 minutes, reducing the intensity level from aerobic to easy.

Running Hill Workout (Runner or Triathlete)

As a warm-up, the athlete runs to the hill while building the intensity from easy to aerobic (this should take about 15 minutes). At the hill, the athlete performs a set of 12 × 2 minutes, running at anaerobic intensity up the hill. The rest interval is the time it takes to walk down the hill. To cool down, the athlete runs home from the hill, descending in intensity from aerobic to easy.

Running Track Workout (Runner or Triathlete)

As a warm-up, the athlete runs for 10 minutes, building in intensity from easy to aerobic. Next, the athlete performs a set of running drills, followed by a set of sprints (optional). The main set is 8 × 800 meters at anaerobic intensity. The rest interval between each 800-meter interval is a 100-meter walk. After completing the workout, the athlete walks for 10 minutes to cool down.

Running Road Workout (Runner or Triathlete)

The athlete should choose a course that allows her to run out and back. An out-and-back is simply a run where the athlete runs out a certain distance (or for a certain amount of time) and then runs back to the starting point. As a warm-up, the athlete runs for 10 minutes, building intensity from easy to aerobic. The main set is 6 × 4 minutes, running at aerobic intensity; between intervals, the athlete rests by walking for 1 minute. At the halfway point of the workout (after the third rest interval), the athlete runs back toward the starting point for the remainder of the workout. The cool-down for this workout is 10 minutes of running with the intensity descending from aerobic to easy.

Running Fartlek Workout (Runner or Triathlete)

This workout is completed on a course that normally takes about an hour to run at an aerobic intensity. The athlete starts the workout by running at an aerobic intensity. During the workout, the athlete completes 10 intervals of 1 to 3 minutes at anaerobic intensity. Each of these intervals is followed by running a minimum of an equal amount of time at aerobic intensity. For example, if an interval at anaerobic intensity is 3 minutes, then the athlete should not start the next anaerobic interval until he has run for at least 3 minutes at aerobic intensity. The workout should be structured so that there is 5 to 10 minutes of running at aerobic intensity at the start and end to allow for a warm-up and cool-down.

AEROBIC WORKOUTS

Moderate-work, moderate-duration workouts (aerobic workouts) are the simplest to execute. For most sports, athletes complete these workouts by simply exercising (e.g., riding or running) for anywhere from 45 to 90 minutes at aerobic intensity. The first 5 to 10 minutes and the last 5 to 10 minutes of these workouts should be used to warm up and cool down. For the warm-up, the athlete builds from easy to aerobic intensity; the athlete does the reverse for the cool-down.

Aerobic workouts are a conservative way to improve endurance. These workouts will boost the endurance of a relative beginner in endurance sport. Aerobic workouts are also effective in the early stages of the training year for most athletes. If an athlete is showing signs of heading toward underrecovery syndrome (i.e., consistent fatigue, poor workouts, reduced appetite, moodiness), performing some aerobic workouts instead of interval workouts will help the athlete maintain balance between workout stress and recovery. For most athletes, a good blend of interval workouts and aerobic workouts is the best complement to long workouts.

Designing training programs is both a science and an art. The science is the easy part. The art is the part that develops with experience. Beginner athletes and coaches need to keep in mind that each athlete is an individual and will react slightly differently when performing a given workout. Many variables may affect how an athlete responds to a training program. Three factors that should be taken into account are the athlete's years of training, current stress levels, and chronological age.

Experience and research have shown that an athlete who has trained consistently will be able to withstand a greater level of training than an athlete who is just starting a training program. The more experienced athlete will usually be able to perform a greater amount of work without incurring negative side effects such as overtraining or inadequate recovery. The more experienced athlete will also be able to handle a greater amount of intensity than the novice athlete. Athletes must avoid falling into the "more is better" strategy of intensity training. The majority of training (as much as 100 percent for the beginning athlete) should be aerobic in nature; even the most experienced athletes should be doing 10 to 15 percent of their work at high intensity. If too much high-intensity work is performed, the athlete will not have adequate recovery. Many athletes—both novice and experienced—make the mistake of training too hard during the low-intensity workouts, which inhibits their ability to go as hard as they should for the higher-intensity work.

Many novice athletes and coaches forget that stress levels hamper an athlete's ability to recover from training. Family, job, and relationships are all potential stressors, as is an athlete's living situation, such as living with a noisy roommate. An athlete or coach needs to be realistic about everything that may affect training. The athlete who is starting a new job, is recently married, or has just moved across the country may respond to training differently than the young and single individual who has no responsibilities other than working and training for competition. The best training programs follow the science of periodized planning, but the athlete or coach should recognize that a plan may need to be adapted or changed depending on how the athlete responds.

Older athletes sometimes require additional rest or recovery in order to achieve the optimal training effect. Older athletes are more likely to have limitations due to previous injuries, aging factors (such as arthritis), disc degeneration, and decreased strength. This doesn't mean that older athletes are unable to compete at high levels. It simply means that younger athletes may have a faster rate of recovery and a greater rate of improvement from training.

Anaerobic and Muscle Endurance Development

Peter Melanson

T his chapter describes the proper exercise techniques for a multitude of free weight and machine exercises. Athletes should be sure to follow the general safety suggestions and lifting guidelines presented at the beginning of this chapter. In addition, they should always follow the manufacturer's safety and usage instructions for each piece of exercise equipment.

Before attempting to perform new exercises, an athlete should always get proper instruction and supervision from a certified strength and conditioning specialist or certified personal trainer (i.e., certified by NSCA). During any free weight and some machine exercises, athletes must make sure that they have proper spotting assistance. Anyone who is considering participating in an exercise program should consult a physician before beginning the program.

LIFTING GUIDELINES

The following guidelines provide basic information that is essential for safe and productive resistance training. Experienced lifters may already know some of this information, but for beginner lifters, understanding these guidelines will be useful whenever they perform resistance training sessions in the weight room.

Technique

Lifters often need to lift a bar or dumbbells off the floor before getting into the starting position for an exercise (e.g., bent-over row, biceps curl, dumbbell flat or incline bench press or fly, upright row, barbell lying triceps extension, stiff-leg deadlift). To avoid excessive strain on the low back, athletes need to place the body in the correct position to lift the weight safely and effectively. Athletes can do this by following these guidelines:

▶ Use the correct stance in relation to the bar or dumbbells and properly grasp the bar or dumbbell handles.

▶ Place the feet between hip- and shoulder-width apart.

▶ Squat down behind the bar or between the dumbbells.

▶ If lifting a bar, position the bar close to the shins and over the balls of the feet, and grasp the bar with a closed grip that is shoulder-width (or slightly wider) apart.

▶ If lifting dumbbells, stand directly between them and grasp the handles with a closed grip and a neutral arm or hand position.

▶ Position the arms outside the knees with the elbows extended.

Before lifting a weight off the floor, athletes must place their body in the correct preparatory position. The following guidelines also describe how the body should be positioned immediately before the first repetition of a power exercise (e.g., snatch, power clean).

▶ The back is flat or slightly arched.

▶ The trapezius is relaxed and slightly stretched, the chest is held up and out, and the scapulae are held together.

▶ The head is in line with the spine or slightly hyperextended.

▶ Body weight is balanced between the middle and balls of the feet, but the heels are in contact with the floor.

▶ The shoulders are over or slightly in front of the bar.

▶ The eyes are focused straight ahead or slightly upward.

Weight Belts

The use of a weight belt can contribute to injury-free training. The decision on whether to use a belt should be based on the type of exercise and the relative load being lifted. Weight belts are most appropriate in the following situations:

▶ During exercises that place stress on the low back (e.g., back squat, front squat, deadlift)

▶ During sets in which near-maximal or maximal loads are being used

The use of a weight belt in these situations may reduce the risk of injuries to the low back—but only when combined with correct exercise technique and proper spotting. Note that some people may have increased blood pressure as a result of wearing a weight belt. Elevated blood pressure is associated with dizziness and fatigue and could result in headaches, fainting, or injury. Additionally, people with hypertension or any preexisting cardiovascular condition should not wear a weight belt because doing so might lead to a heart attack or stroke.

GENERAL SAFETY SUGGESTIONS

Athletes should follow these guidelines to ensure safe exercise technique:

- Perform power and explosive exercises in an area that is clean, dry, flat, well marked, and free of obstacles and people (e.g., on a lifting platform). This guideline also applies to other complex nonpower exercises such as the lunge, deadlift, and step-up. If a repetition in a power or explosive exercise cannot be completed, the athlete should push forward on the bar to move the body backward and then let the bar fall to the floor. Athletes should not attempt to "save" a missed or failed repetition for this type of exercise.

- Check to see if there is sufficient floor-to-ceiling space before performing exercises that finish with the bar overhead. Athletes should use a bar with revolving sleeves, especially for the power and explosive exercises.

- For the front squat and back squat, use a squat or power rack with the supporting pins or hooks set to position the bar at armpit height. This setting should also be used when the preferred method for an exercise is to begin or end with the bar at shoulder height (rather than begin or end with the bar on the floor).

- When lifting the bar up and out of the supporting pins or hooks of a squat or power rack in preparation for an exercise, always step backward at the beginning of the set and step forward at the end of the set. The athlete should not walk backward to return the bar to the rack. This is a good safety practice that reduces the potential for a misstep when fatigued.

- When using free weights, always use collars and locks to secure the weight plates on the bar.

- For machine exercises, be sure to fully insert the selectorized pin or key (usually L or T shaped) into the weight stack.

- A spotter should assist for safety during free weight exercises.

Snatch-Grip Hand Placement

The snatch-grip hand placement on the bar is wider than it is for other exercises. To help an athlete estimate the proper width of the grip, have the athlete extend an arm laterally and parallel to the floor; then measure the distance from the edge of the knuckles of that arm (the athlete should clench the fist) to the outside edge of the opposite shoulder (see figure 6.1). Alternatively, the lifter's grip width can be estimated by measuring the elbow-to-elbow distance when the upper arms are abducted directly out from the sides and parallel to the floor (see figure 6.2). This distance is the space between the hands when they are grasping the bar. If necessary, this spacing can be modified depending on shoulder flexibility and arm length. In this grip, the hands face backward in a pronated position.

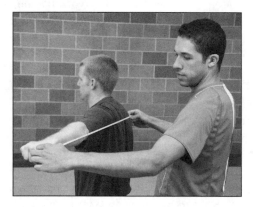

Figure 6.1 Option 1 for estimating the proper width of the snatch grip.

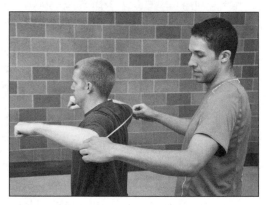

Figure 6.2 Option 2 for estimating the proper width of the snatch grip.

Grips

Different types of grips are used for different exercises. Two basic positions are used for placing the hands on the bar. In the pronated position, the bar is gripped with the palm facing backward. A pronated grip is used for almost all exercises that require the weight to be lifted above the head. In the supinated hand position, the palm is facing forward when grasping the bar. When the thumb is wrapped around the fingers that are grasping the bar, this is referred to as a closed grip (see figure 6.3a). On the rare occasion when the bar is gripped with the thumb in line with the fingers, this is referred to as an open grip. An open grip is less secure than a closed grip and will increase the risk of accidents. For the Olympic lifts, a variation of the closed grip—called the hook grip (see figure 6.3b)—or a clean and jerk grip can be used to ensure optimal performance.

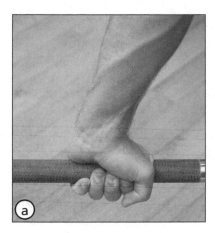 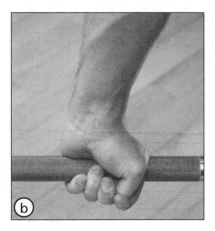

Figure 6.3   The *(a)* closed pronated grip and the *(b)* hook grip.

TYPES OF EXERCISES

This chapter provides information on three main types of resistance exercises: Olympic lifts, lower-body lifts, and upper-body lifts. Olympic lifts use large muscle groups and involve multiple body parts being worked at the same time. These exercises help an athlete develop coordination, strength, and power. In a given workout, Olympic lifts should be done first because performing these lifts correctly requires the most concentration and skill. Athletes who are not familiar with Olympic lifting should seek out an experienced lifting coach to ensure that they are performing the exercises safely.

Some athletes may not have access to a gym with an Olympic lifting platform, or they may prefer to train at home so they can avoid the time commitment required to regularly travel to a gym. Many of the upper- and lower-body exercises can be performed with dumbbells, which are relatively inexpensive to purchase. Many athletes purchase a flat bench and a set of adjustable dumbbells. The cost of these items is less than the cost of participating in one or two endurance races (especially if the items are purchased used), and the equipment will last a lifetime.

POWER CLEAN

The athlete stands with the feet between hip- and shoulder-width apart; the toes are pointed forward or slightly outward. The athlete squats and grasps the bar with the hands slightly wider than the shoulders (and outside the knees) using a closed, pronated grip. He straightens the elbows and positions the body so the back is flat or slightly arched (photo *a*); the chest is up, the shoulders are over the bar, and the eyes are focused forward or slightly up.

1. The athlete forcefully extends the hips and knees to lift the bar, keeping the torso-to-floor angle constant by maintaining a flat-back position. He keeps the elbows fully extended and keeps the bar as close to the shins as possible.

2. As the bar rises to just above the knees, the athlete forcefully extends the hips and knees and also extends the ankles (plantar flexion). He keeps the bar as close to the body as possible. The athlete's back remains flat, and the elbows are pointing out to the sides. The athlete keeps the shoulders over the bar and the elbows extended for as long as possible.

3. When the ankle, knee, and hip reach full extension (triple extension), the athlete shrugs the shoulders upward with the elbows still fully extended. As the shoulders reach their highest elevation, the athlete flexes the elbows to begin pulling the body under the bar. He continues pulling with the arms high as long as possible. The torso is erect, the head is erect or tilted slightly back, and the feet may lose contact with the floor (photo *b*). After the lower body has fully extended, the athlete pulls the body under the bar and rotates the arms around and under the bar. Simultaneously, he flexes the hips and knees to a quarter-squat position.

4. Once the arms are under the bar, the athlete lifts the elbows so that the upper arms are parallel to the floor. He racks the bar across the front of the clavicles and anterior deltoids. When the athlete catches the bar, the torso is nearly erect, the shoulders are slightly ahead of the buttocks, the head is in a neutral position, and the feet are flat.

5. After gaining control and balance, the athlete stands up by extending the hips and knees to a fully erect position (photo *c*).

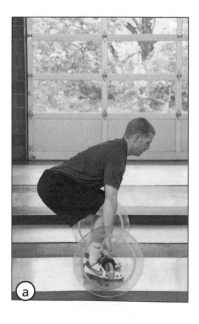
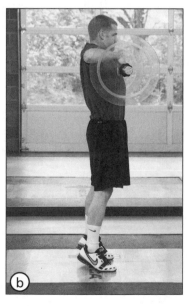
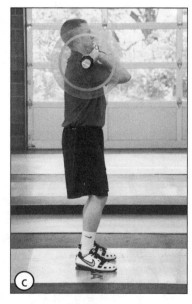

a

b

c

HANG POWER CLEAN

The athlete begins in a hip-width stance, holding the bar with a closed, pronated grip. He holds the bar in front of the body, touching the thighs. The scapulae are tightly squeezed together. The athlete lowers the bar to just above the knee by pushing the hips back so that the bar slides down the front of the thighs (photo *a*). He positions the body with the knees slightly bent, the back flat or slightly arched, and the chest up. The shoulders are over or slightly in front of the bar, and the eyes are focused straight ahead or slightly upward.

1. The athlete quickly and explosively performs triple extension in a jumping action while maintaining a flat-back position. The elbows are pointed out, and the athlete keeps the bar as close to the body as possible. He keeps the shoulders over the bar and the elbows extended for as long as possible.

2. When the full triple extension is reached, the athlete rapidly shrugs the shoulders upward with the elbows still fully extended. As the shoulders reach their highest elevation, the athlete flexes the elbows to begin pulling the body under the bar. He continues to pull with the arms high for as long as possible. Because of the explosive nature of this phase, the feet may lose contact with the floor. The torso is erect, and the head is tilted slightly back.

3. After the lower body has fully extended, the athlete pulls the body under the bar and rotates the arms around and under the bar while flexing the hips and knees into a quarter squat (photo *b*).

4. Once the arms are under the bar, the athlete lifts the elbows so that the upper arms are parallel to the floor. He racks the bar across the front of the clavicles and anterior deltoids. When the athlete catches the bar, the torso is nearly erect, the shoulders are slightly ahead of the buttocks, the head is in a neutral position, and the feet are flat.

5. When balanced, the athlete stands up by fully extending the hips and knees (photo *c*).

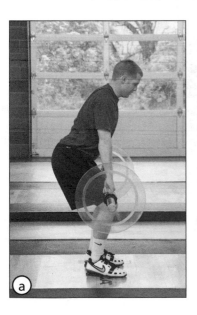
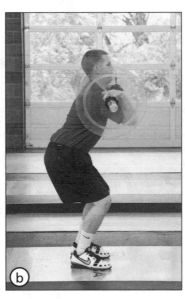
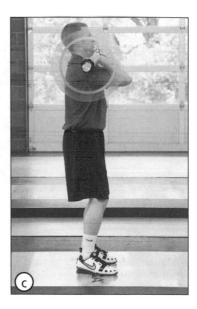

POWER CLEAN AND PUSH PRESS

The athlete follows the directions for the power clean (provided earlier in this chapter; photo *a*). Once he has finished the power clean movement, the athlete continues with the push press described here.

1. The athlete resets the feet in a hip-width position. He squats at a slow to moderate speed to move the bar in a straight path downward. The athlete should continue the squat to a depth that does not exceed a quarter squat, the catch position of the power clean, or 10 percent of the athlete's height (photo *b*). The feet are flat on the floor, the torso is erect, and the upper arms are parallel to the floor.

2. On reaching the lowest position of the squat, the athlete quickly extends the hips and knees and then the elbows to move the bar overhead.

3. After the hips and knees are fully extended and the bar is overhead, the athlete flexes the hips and knees and simultaneously extends the elbows fully. He catches the bar overhead at the moment that the bar reaches its highest position. The torso

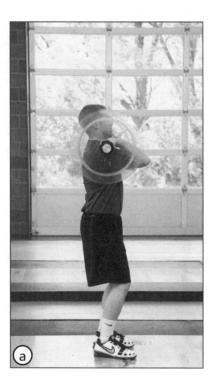

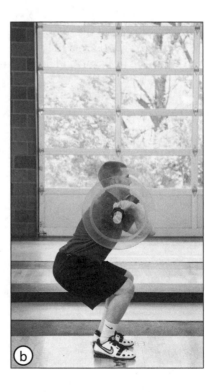

is erect, the head is in a neutral position, the feet are flat on the floor, and the bar is slightly behind the head (photo c).

4. The athlete lowers the bar by gradually allowing a controlled descent of the bar to the shoulders. He simultaneously flexes the hips and knees to cushion the impact of the bar on the shoulders.

If the athlete wants to practice the push press movement by itself before combining it with the power clean, he can do so in a squat rack. The athlete grasps the bar using a closed, pronated grip with the hands slightly wider than shoulder width. He steps under the bar with the feet facing forward and positioned hip-width apart. The athlete places the bar on top of the anterior deltoids and clavicles (photo d). He extends the hips and knees to lift the bar off the supports. He then positions the feet hip-width apart (or slightly wider) with the toes pointed slightly outward.

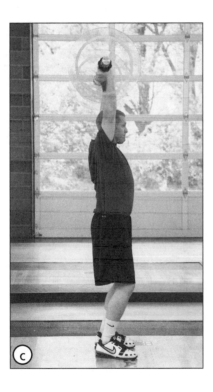

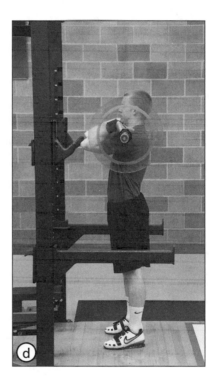

POWER CLEAN AND PRESS

The athlete follows the directions for the power clean (on page 90; photo *a*). Once he has finished the power clean movement and is standing up, the athlete continues with the press portion described here.

1. Using the upper body, the athlete pushes the barbell directly overhead until the elbows are locked out. He pauses with the arms fully extended, maintaining a rigid torso position and a slight bend in the knees and hips (photo *b*).

2. The athlete lowers the bar by gradually allowing a controlled descent of the bar to the shoulders. He simultaneously flexes the hips and knees to cushion the impact of the bar on the shoulders.

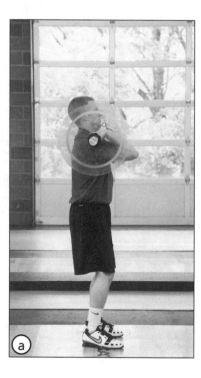
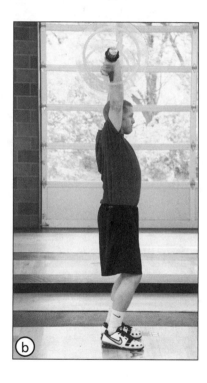

POWER CLEAN AND PUSH JERK

The athlete follows the directions for the power clean (on page 90; photo *a*). Once he has finished the power clean movement and is standing up, the athlete continues with the push jerk.

1. The athlete squats at a slow to moderate speed to move the bar in a straight path downward. He should continue the squat to a depth that does not exceed a quarter squat, or 10 percent of the athlete's height. The feet are flat on the floor, the torso is erect, and the upper arms are parallel to the floor.

2. The athlete reverses the movement by quickly and explosively extending the hips and knees and then the elbows to move the bar overhead.

3. After the hips and knees are fully extended and the bar is overhead, the athlete quickly flexes the hips and knees to a quarter-squat position while extending the elbows to catch the bar as it reaches its highest position (photo *b*). The torso is erect, the head is in a neutral position, the feet are flat, and the bar is slightly behind the head.

4. The athlete lowers the bar by gradually allowing a controlled descent of the bar to the shoulders. He simultaneously flexes the hips and knees to cushion the impact of the bar on the shoulders.

If an athlete wants to practice the push jerk movement by itself before combining it with the power clean, he can do so in a squat rack.

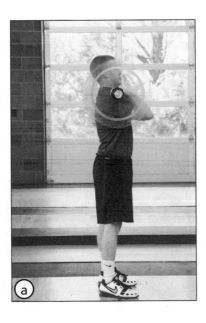
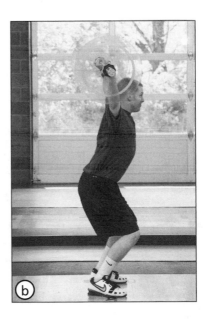

CLEAN PULL FROM FLOOR

The athlete stands with the feet straight ahead or slightly outward between hip- and shoulder-width apart. He squats and grasps the bar using a closed, pronated grip with the hands positioned slightly wider than shoulder width (and outside the knees); the elbows are extended. The back is flat or slightly arched, and the chest is held up (photo *a*). The shoulders are over or slightly in front of the bar, and the scapulae are tightly squeezed together.

1. The athlete lifts the bar off the floor by extending the hips and knees. The torso-to-floor angle should remain constant, and the athlete maintains a flat-back position. The elbows are fully extended, and the shoulders are over or slightly ahead of the bar. As the bar is raised, the athlete keeps it as close to the shins as possible.

2. As the bar rises to just above the knees (photo *b*), the athlete forcefully jumps upward by triple extension. He keeps the bar as close to the body as possible, with the back flat and the elbows pointing out. The athlete keeps the shoulders over the bar and keeps the elbows extended.

3. After full triple extension, the athlete rapidly shrugs the shoulders with the elbows extended (photo *c*). Because of the explosive nature of this phase, the feet may lose contact with the floor.

4. After the lower body has fully extended, the athlete returns to the starting position. He should safely land on the floor by flexing the hips and knees to cushion the impact of the bar pulling on the shoulders and spine.

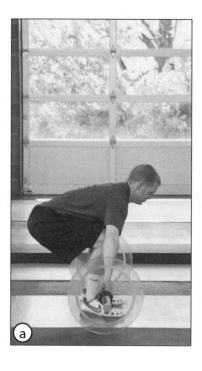
(a)

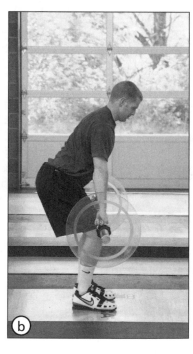
(b)

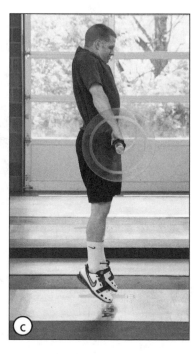
(c)

CLEAN PULL FROM KNEE-HIGH BLOCKS

The athlete begins in a hip-width stance while grasping the bar with a closed, pronated grip. The bar is in front of the body and is sitting on a pair of blocks (or scoops) at knee height. (This exercise can also be performed using blocks at mid-thigh height.) The bar should be touching the top of the knee. The athlete positions the body with the knees slightly bent, the back flat or slightly arched, and the chest held up and out (photo *a*). The shoulders are over or slightly in front of the bar, the scapulae are tightly squeezed together, and the eyes are focused straight ahead, in front, or slightly upward.

1. The athlete executes the lift by quickly and explosively extending the hips, knees, and ankles in a jumping action. He keeps the bar as close to the body as possible. The back is flat, and the elbows are pointing out to the side. The athlete keeps the shoulders over the bar and keeps the elbows extended.

2. When the lower-body joints reach full extension, the athlete rapidly shrugs the shoulders upward with the elbows still fully extended (photo *b*). He should not allow the elbows to bend. Because of the explosive nature of this phase, the feet may lose contact with the floor. The torso is erect, and the head is tilted slightly back.

3. After the lower body has fully extended, the athlete returns to the starting position. He safely lands on the floor and drops the bar onto the blocks or scoops.

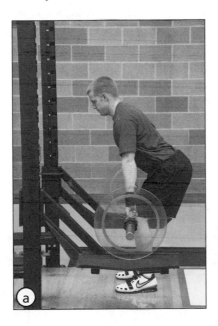 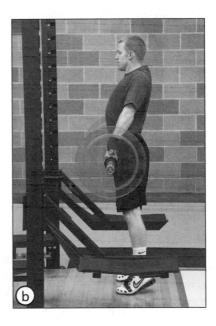

POWER SNATCH

The athlete stands with the feet pointed slightly out and positioned between hip- and shoulder-width apart. He squats and grasps the bar using a closed, pronated, snatch-width grip (photo a). The athlete positions the body with the back flat or slightly arched, the trapezius relaxed and slightly stretched, and the chest held up and out. The heels are in contact with the floor, and the shoulders are over or slightly in front of the bar.

1. The athlete lifts the bar by extending the hips and knees while maintaining the flat-back position; the torso-to-floor angle should remain constant. The elbows stay fully extended, and the shoulders remain over or slightly ahead of the bar. The athlete keeps the bar as close to the shins as possible.

2. As the bar rises to just above the knees, the athlete forcefully jumps, performing triple extension. He keeps the bar as close to the body as possible. The back stays flat, the elbows are extended and pointing out, and the shoulders are over the bar.

3. After reaching full triple extension, the athlete rapidly shrugs the shoulders upward with the elbows still fully extended. As the shoulders reach their highest elevation, the athlete flexes the elbows to begin pulling the body under the bar (photo b). He continues to pull with the arms for as long as possible. Because of the explosive nature of this phase, the feet may lose contact with the floor.

4. After the lower body has fully extended, the athlete pulls the body beneath the bar and rotates the hands around and under the bar. Simultaneously, the athlete flexes the hips and knees to a quarter-squat position.

5. Once the body is under the bar, the athlete catches the bar over or slightly behind the head with fully extended elbows, a neutral head position, and flat feet (photo c). After gaining control and balance, the athlete stands up by extending the hips and knees to a fully erect position. He stabilizes the bar overhead.

6. The athlete lowers the bar by gradually allowing a controlled descent of the bar to the thighs. He simultaneously flexes the hips and knees to cushion the impact of the bar on the thighs.

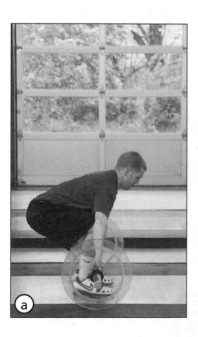

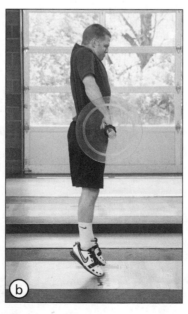

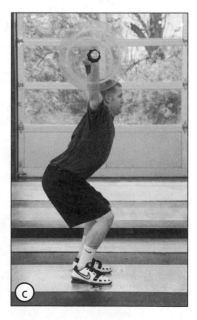

HANG POWER SNATCH

The athlete begins in a hip-width stance while grasping the bar with a snatch grip; the bar is touching the thighs (photo *a*). The athlete's scapulae are tightly squeezed together. The athlete positions the body with the knees slightly bent, the back flat or slightly arched, and the chest held up. The shoulders are over or slightly in front of the bar.

1. The athlete executes the lift by performing triple extension in a jumping action. He keeps the bar as close to the body as possible. The back remains flat, the elbows are extended and pointing out, and the shoulders are over the bar.

2. After reaching full triple extension, the athlete shrugs the shoulders upward with the elbows still fully extended.

3. As the shoulders reach their highest elevation, the athlete flexes the elbows to begin pulling the body under the bar. He continues to pull with the arms high for as long as possible. Because of the explosive nature of this phase, the feet may slightly lose contact with the floor (photo *b*).

4. After the lower body has fully extended, the athlete pulls the body beneath the bar and rotates the hands around and under the bar. Simultaneously, the athlete flexes the hips and knees to a quarter-squat position.

5. Once the body is under the bar, the athlete catches the bar over or slightly behind the head with fully extended elbows, a neutral head position, and flat feet (photo *c*). After gaining control and balance, the athlete stands up by extending the hips and knees to a fully erect position. He stabilizes the bar overhead.

6. The athlete lowers the bar by gradually allowing a controlled descent of the bar to the thighs. He simultaneously flexes the hips and knees to cushion the impact of the bar on the thighs.

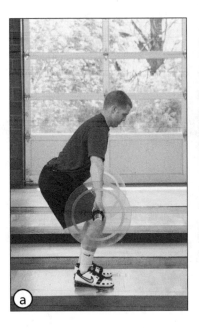
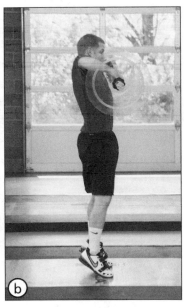
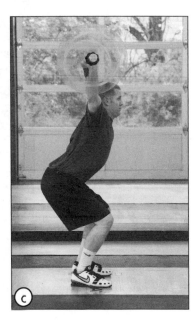

SNATCH PULL FROM KNEE-HIGH BLOCKS

The athlete begins in a hip-width stance while grasping the bar with a closed, pronated snatch grip. The bar is in front of the body and is sitting on a pair of blocks (or scoops) at knee height. The bar should be touching the top of the kneecap. The athlete positions the body with the knees slightly bent, the back flat or slightly arched, and the chest held up and out (photo a). The shoulders are over or slightly in front of the bar, the scapulae are tightly squeezed together, and the eyes are focused straight ahead, in front, or slightly upward.

1. The athlete executes the lift by quickly and explosively extending the hips, knees, and ankles in a jumping action. He keeps the bar as close to the body as possible. The back remains flat, and the elbows are pointing out to the side. The athlete keeps the shoulders over the bar and keeps the elbows extended for as long as possible.

2. When the lower-body joints reach full extension, the athlete rapidly shrugs the shoulders upward with the elbows still fully extended (photo b). He should not allow the elbows to bend. Because of the explosive nature of this phase, the feet may lose contact with the floor. The torso is erect, and the head may be tilted back slightly.

3. After the lower body has fully extended, the athlete returns to the starting position. He safely lands on the floor and drops the bar onto the blocks or scoops.

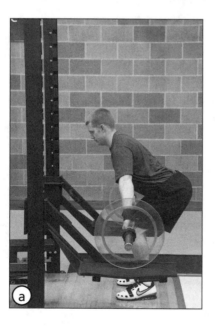 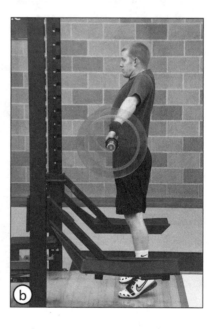

POWER SNATCH PLUS OVERHEAD SQUAT

1. The athlete follows the directions for the power snatch (through step 5 as described on page 98; photo *a*).

2. The athlete then readjusts the feet to proper squatting position. He slowly lowers himself in a squatting motion by sitting back with the hips (photo *b*) until the top of the thighs are parallel to the floor (photo *c*). The athlete must be sure to keep the torso in a rigid and erect position while maintaining good balance.

3. The athlete then extends the legs at the hips and knees, returning to the starting position while maintaining a rigid torso with the bar overhead.

4. The athlete lowers the bar from the overhead position by gradually reducing the muscular tension of the shoulders.

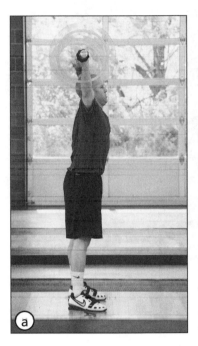
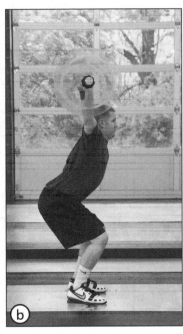
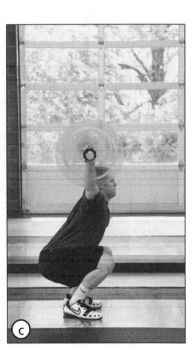

SQUAT

The athlete assumes a shoulder-width stance, holding the barbell on top of the scapulae and trapezius (photo *a*). The hands are slightly wider than the shoulders. The toes may be pointed outward slightly.

1. Keeping the torso erect, the athlete squats by sitting back with the hips until the top of the thighs are parallel to the floor (photo *b*).
2. The athlete then extends the legs at the hips and knees to return to the starting position.

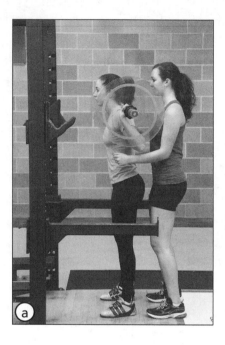 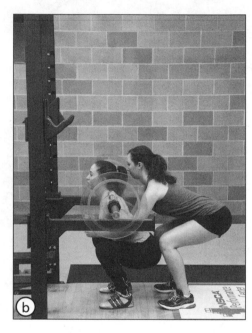

FRONT SQUAT

The athlete assumes a shoulder-width stance, with the toes pointing out slightly. She positions the elbows as high in front of the body as possible so that the barbell rests on the front of the shoulder (photo *a*). The hands are slightly wider than the shoulders.

1. Keeping the torso erect, the athlete squats by lowering the body at the knees and hips until the top of the thighs are parallel to the floor (photo *b*). She keeps the elbows elevated as high as possible.

2. The athlete then extends the legs at the hips and knees to return to the starting position.

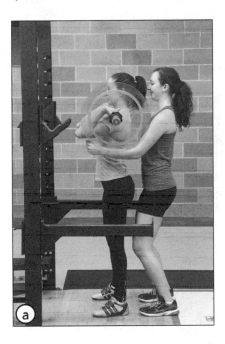 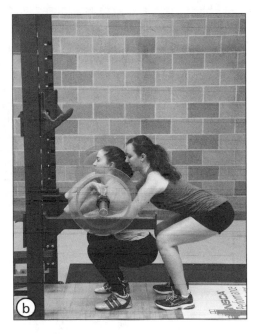

SQUAT AND PRESS

The athlete begins in a shoulder-width stance, holding the barbell on top of the scapulae and trapezius (photo *a*). The hands are slightly wider than the shoulders. The toes may be pointed outward slightly.

1. Keeping the torso erect, the athlete squats by sitting back with the hips until the top of the thighs are parallel to the floor.

2. The athlete then extends the legs at the hips and knees to return to the starting position.

3. Without stopping, the athlete pushes the barbell directly overhead until the elbows are locked out (photo *b*). He pauses with the arms fully extended, maintaining a rigid torso position. The knees and hips may be slightly bent.

4. The athlete allows the elbows to slowly flex, lowering the bar to the shoulder and trapezius. He uses the knees as shock absorbers to catch the bar.

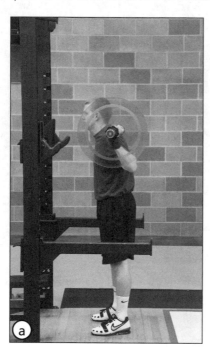 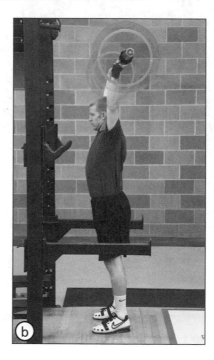

OVERHEAD SQUAT

The athlete begins in a shoulder-width stance, holding the barbell overhead with a snatch grip. He pushes the head through so the arms are behind the ears in a locked-out position (photo *a*). The toes may be pointed outward slightly.

1. The athlete squats by sitting back with the hips until the top of the thighs are parallel to the floor (photo *b*). He keeps the torso in a rigid and erect position while maintaining good balance.

2. The athlete then extends the legs at the hips and knees to return to the starting position.

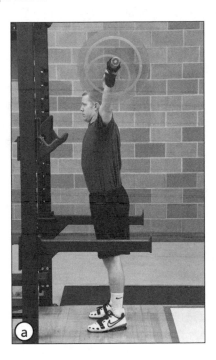 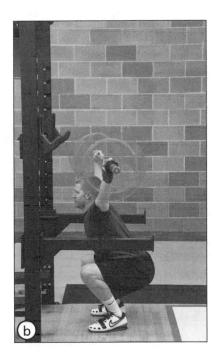

SPEED SQUAT

The athlete begins in a shoulder-width stance, holding the barbell on top of the scapulae and trapezius (photo a). The hands are slightly wider than the shoulders. The toes may be pointed outward slightly. The athlete performs this movement at an accelerated pace from a normal squat, but not so fast that form is sacrificed. The athlete must maintain proper form and ensure that the bar does not come off the shoulders and that the feet do not leave the ground during the upward portion of this exercise.

1. Keeping the torso erect, the athlete squats by sitting back with the hips until the top of the thighs are parallel to the floor (photo b).
2. The athlete then extends the legs at the hips and knees to return to the starting position.

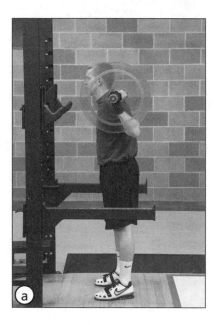 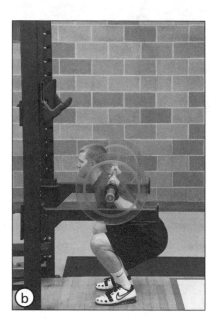

SINGLE-LEG LUNGE

The athlete starts in a shoulder-width stance and then places the top of one foot on top of a 12- to 18-inch (30.5 to 45.7 cm) box or bench behind him. He holds a barbell on top of the scapulae (photo *a*).

1. The athlete flexes at the knee and hip of the supporting leg until the top of the front thigh is parallel to the floor (photo *b*).The back knee should be about 1 inch (2.5 cm) above the floor. The athlete should keep the front foot flat on the floor and keep the knee in line with the second and third toe of the lead foot. He should not let the knee extend forward excessively past the toes.

2. The athlete pushes through the supporting leg and returns to the starting position.

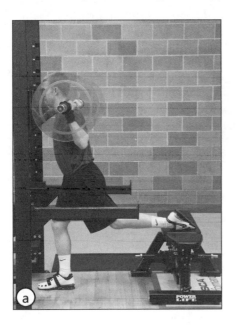
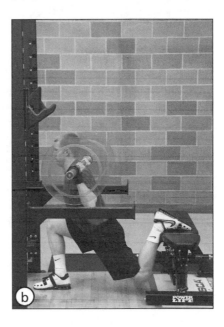

LUNGE (BARBELL OR DUMBBELL)

The athlete starts in a shoulder-width stance. She holds a barbell on top of the scapulae (photo a) or holds a pair of dumbbells (one in each hand) at the sides of the body.

1. The athlete begins by stepping forward with one leg. She must make sure that the step is not so large that she loses her balance.
2. When the entire foot makes contact with the floor, the athlete flexes at the knees and hips until the top of the front thigh is parallel to the floor (photo b). The back knee should be about 1 inch (2.5 cm) above the floor. The athlete should keep the front foot flat on the floor and keep the knee in line with the second and third toe of the lead foot. She should not let the knee extend forward excessively past the toes.
3. The athlete forcefully pushes back with the front leg to return to the starting position.
4. The athlete repeats the movement with the other leg.

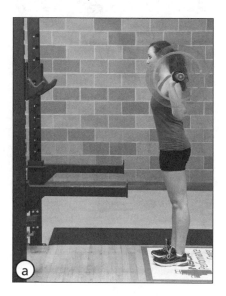 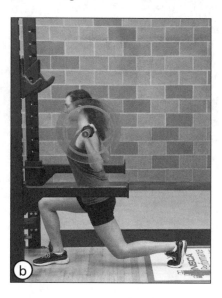

REVERSE LUNGE

The athlete starts in a shoulder-width stance. She holds a barbell on top of the scapulae or holds a pair of dumbbells (one in each hand) at the sides of the body (photo *a*).

1. The athlete begins by stepping backward with one leg. She must make sure that the step is not so large that she loses her balance.
2. When the foot makes contact with the floor, the athlete flexes the front knee and hip until the top of the front thigh is parallel to the floor (photo *b*). The back knee should be about 1 inch (2.5 cm) above the floor. The athlete should keep the front foot flat on the floor and keep the knee in line with the second and third toes of the lead foot. She should not let the knee extend forward past the toes.
3. Using the back leg, the athlete pushes back up, extending the hip and knee of the front leg to return to the starting position.
4. The athlete repeats the movement with the other leg.

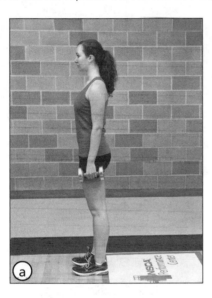 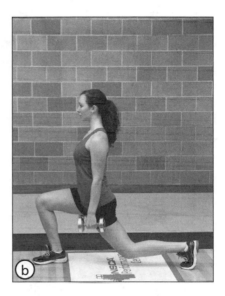

STEP-UP (BARBELL OR DUMBBELL)

The athlete places the lead foot on top of a box; the box should be high enough so that the knee is at a 90-degree angle. The athlete positions a barbell on the upper back (photo *a*) or holds a pair of dumbbells (one in each hand) at the sides of the body. With one foot on top of the box, the athlete shifts the weight to the lead leg to prevent herself from pushing off the floor with the trail leg. (She curls up the toes of the trail leg to also help avoid pushing off with this leg.)

1. The athlete extends the hip and knee of the lead leg to a standing position on top of the box. She should keep the torso erect and avoid bending forward at the hips.
2. The athlete brings the trail leg up to the box and positions the foot parallel to the lead foot (photo *b*).
3. The athlete steps down with the trail leg, moving back to the starting position.
4. The athlete repeats this movement for the desired number of repetitions and then switches legs.

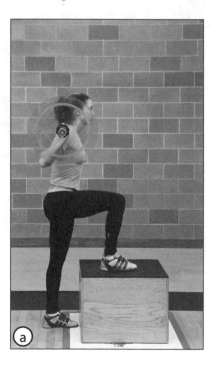
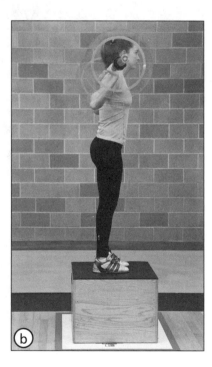

STEP-UP DRIVE-THROUGH (BARBELL OR DUMBBELL)

The athlete places the lead foot on top of a box; the box should be high enough so that the knee is at a 90-degree angle. The athlete positions a barbell on the upper back, creating a shelf with the scapulae for the bar (photo *a*), or holds a pair of dumbbells (one in each hand) at the sides of the body. With one foot on top of the box, the athlete shifts the weight to the lead leg to prevent herself from pushing off the floor with the trail leg. (She curls up the toes of the trail leg to also help avoid pushing off with this leg.)

1. The athlete extends the hip and knee of the lead leg to a standing position on top of the box. She should keep the torso erect and avoid bending forward at the hips.
2. The athlete brings the trail leg up, driving the knee upward to about a chest-high position (photo *b*).
3. The athlete steps down with the trail leg, moving back to the starting position.
4. The athlete repeats this movement for the desired number of repetitions and then switches legs.

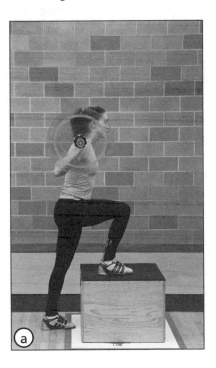 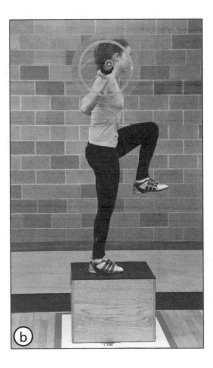

GOOD MORNING

The athlete grasps the bar with a closed, pronated grip. The feet are parallel to each other and positioned hip-width apart. The athlete places the bar on the upper back and shoulders above the posterior deltoids at the base of the neck (using a grip that is slightly wider than shoulder width; photo *a*). He should lift the elbows up to create a shelf for the bar using the upper back and shoulder muscles. The athlete holds the chest up and out and tilts the head slightly up.

1. The athlete begins the exercise by hinging at the hips. The buttocks should move straight back during the descent. The athlete maintains a flat-back and high-elbow position (photo *b*); he should not round the upper back. The bar should be slightly behind the toes; the athlete should not allow the heels to rise off the floor. The athlete keeps the knees slightly flexed during the descent. He continues the downward movement until the torso is approximately parallel to the floor.

2. The athlete raises the bar by extending the hips. He keeps the back flat and the knees slightly flexed during the ascent. The athlete continues extending the hips to reach the starting position.

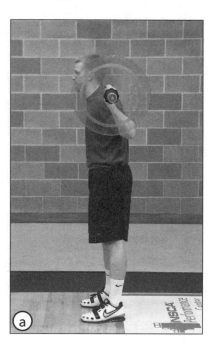

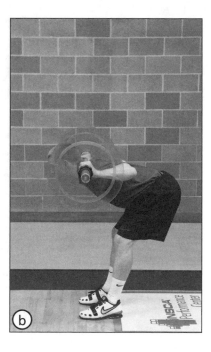

CLEAN-GRIP ROMANIAN DEADLIFT (RDL)

The athlete stands with the feet hip-width apart. Using a clean grip, the athlete holds a barbell against the front of the thighs. He unlocks the knees so there is a slight bend and maintains the slight bend throughout the duration of the exercise (photo *a*). The athlete should squeeze the scapulae together so that the shoulders do not round during the movement.

1. The athlete begins by pushing the hips back and sliding the bar down the front of the thighs. He keeps the torso rigid and keeps the lower back flat or slightly arched (photo *b*). The athlete lowers until the bar is about 1 or 2 inches (2.5 to 5.0 cm) below the kneecap (or until proper form can no longer be maintained).
2. The athlete returns to the starting position, keeping the shoulders back, the back arched, the head up, and the bar in contact with the legs at all times.

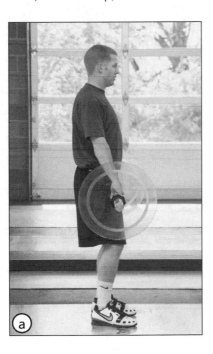
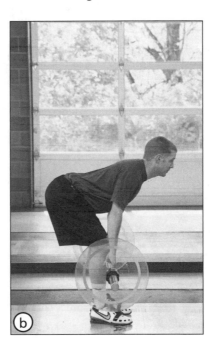

LEG CURL (MACHINE)

Machines may differ, so athletes should be sure to read and understand the directions printed on the equipment being used. To get into position, the athlete presses the hips and torso firmly against the pads. She places the ankle behind and in contact with the roller pad (photo *a*). The thighs should be parallel to each other, and the knees should be slightly off the bottom edge of the thigh pad. The athlete aligns the knees with the axis of the machine. She grasps the handles or the sides of the chest pad.

1. The athlete raises the roller pad by fully flexing the knee (photo *b*). She keeps the torso stationary and keeps the hips and torso firmly pressed against the pads.

2. The athlete allows the knee to slowly extend back to the starting position. The athlete should not forcefully lock out the knee.

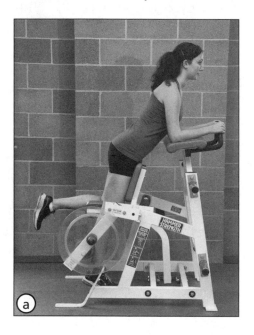 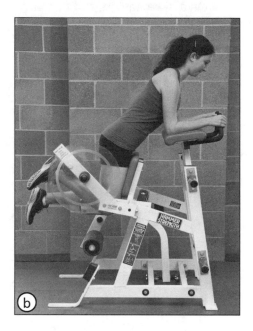

DUMBBELL CALF RAISE

The athlete stands with both feet side by side near the edge of a raised surface—such as a box, bench, or stair. The athlete holds a dumbbell at each side (photo a). (This exercise can also be done alternating legs. In this case, the athlete holds a dumbbell on the side of the working leg. If necessary, he can hold on to something with the other hand for stability.)

1. The athlete rises up on the toes as high as possible while keeping the knees extended or just slightly bent (photo b).
2. The athlete returns to the starting position.

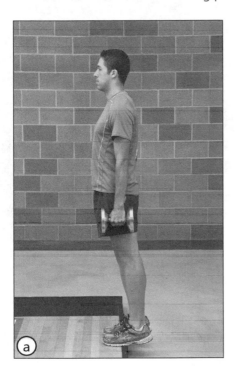
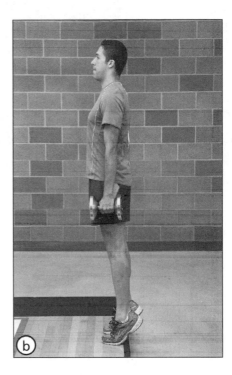

BARBELL CALF RAISE

The athlete stands with both feet side by side near the edge of a solid raised surface while holding the barbell on top of the scapulae and trapezius (photo *a*). The hands are positioned slightly wider than the shoulders.

1. The athlete rises up on the toes as high as possible while keeping the knees extended or just slightly bent (photo *b*).
2. The athlete returns to the starting position.

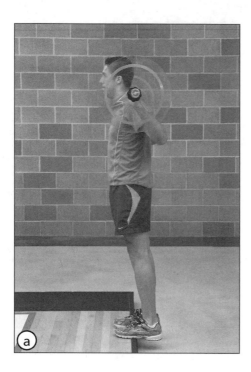 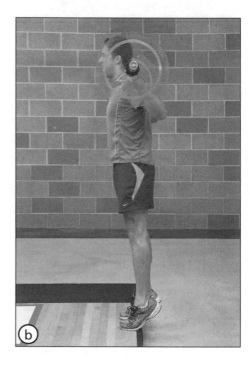

SPLIT-SQUAT JUMP

The athlete begins in a split stance, holding small weights with the arms hanging straight down at the sides. The heel of the rear foot is off the floor, and the front foot is flat.

1. The athlete lowers the body into a split-squat position (photo *a*). She then explodes upward with the front leg to gain vertical height while maintaining control of the weights and keeping the arms at the side of the body (photo *b*).
2. On landing, the athlete should stick the position, demonstrating body control.
3. The athlete repeats the jump for the desired number of repetitions and then switches legs.

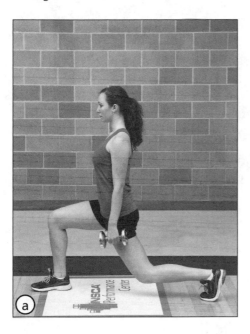
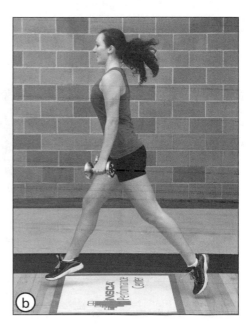

BARBELL BENCH PRESS

Using a flat bench, the athlete assumes a position with the standard five points of contact: The head, shoulders, and glutes are in contact with the bench, and both feet are on the floor. The athlete uses an overhand (pronated) grip on the bar, with the hands positioned slightly wider than shoulder width. The athlete lifts the bar off the rack until it is directly over the chest (photo *a*).

1. In a controlled manner, the athlete lowers the bar to the chest.

2. The athlete touches the bar against the chest (photo *b*) and then pushes the weight back to the starting position.

3. The athlete repeats this movement for the desired number of repetitions, returning the barbell to the rack on completion of the final repetition.

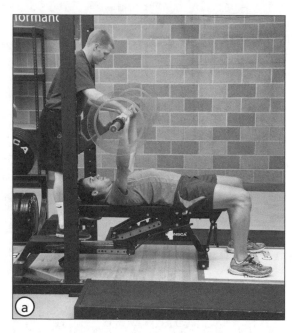

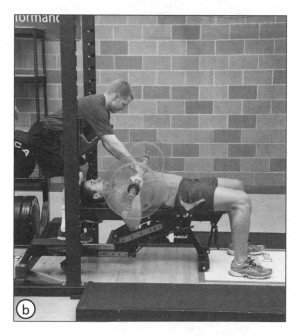

DUMBBELL BENCH PRESS

Using a flat bench, the athlete begins with a dumbbell in each hand. He lies back on the bench using the standard five points of contact. The athlete places each dumbbell at shoulder width and at just above armpit height (photo *a*).

1. The athlete presses the dumbbells up toward the ceiling until the arms are fully extended (photo *b*).
2. The athlete then lowers the dumbbells to their starting position.

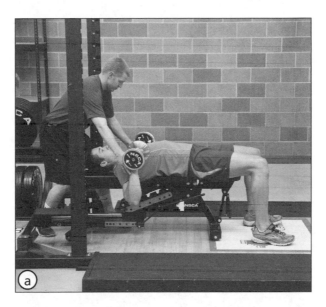

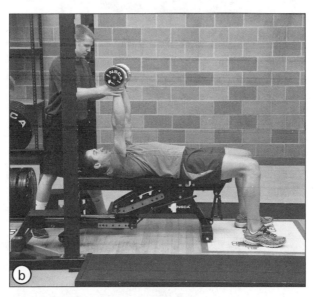

BARBELL INCLINE BENCH PRESS

Using an incline bench, the athlete assumes a position with the standard five points of contact. The athlete uses an overhand grip on the bar, with the hands positioned slightly wider than shoulder width. The eyes are lined up directly with the bar. The athlete lifts the bar off the rack until it is positioned directly over the top of the chest (photo *a*).

1. In a controlled manner, the athlete lowers the bar to the top part of the chest.
2. The athlete touches the bar against the chest (photo *b*) and then pushes the weight back to the starting position.
3. The athlete repeats this movement for the desired number of repetitions, returning the barbell to the rack on completion of the final repetition.

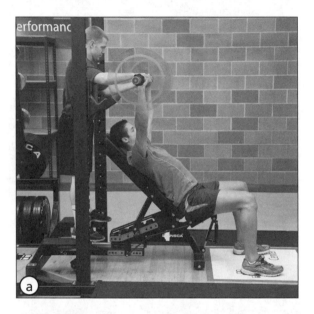

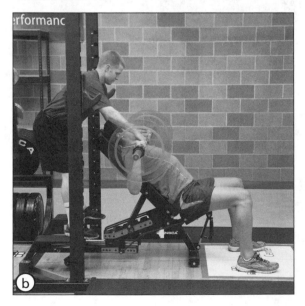

DUMBBELL INCLINE BENCH PRESS

Using an incline bench, the athlete begins with a dumbbell in each hand; he lies back on the bench using the standard five points of contact. The athlete places each dumbbell at shoulder width and at just above armpit height (photo *a*).

1. The athlete presses the dumbbells up toward the ceiling until the arms are fully extended (photo *b*).
2. The athlete then lowers the dumbbells to their starting position.

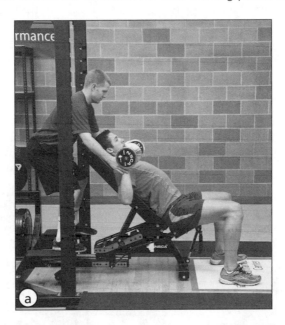

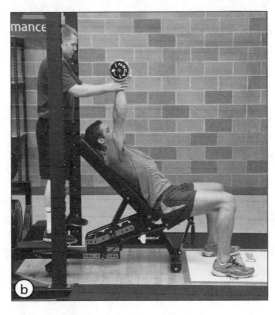

BENCH PRESS WITH MEDICINE BALL TOSS

In this exercise, the athlete performs a bench press followed by a medicine ball toss from the floor. Using a flat bench, the athlete assumes a position with the standard five points of contact. The athlete uses an overhand grip on the bar, with the hands positioned slightly wider than shoulder width. The eyes are lined up directly with the bar. The athlete lifts the bar off the rack until it is directly over the chest.

1. In a controlled manner, the athlete lowers the bar to the chest.
2. The athlete touches the bar against the chest and then pushes the weight back to the starting position.
3. The athlete repeats this movement for the desired number of repetitions, returning the barbell to the rack on completion of the final repetition.
4. After the final repetition of the bench press, the athlete immediately sits on the floor and picks up a medicine ball. The athlete sits with the torso at about a 60-degree angle, the knees bent, and the feet flat on the floor (photo a).
5. The athlete holds the medicine ball at chest level and uses both hands to throw it forward as far as possible (photo b). If the athlete does not have a partner, he can throw the medicine ball against a wall.

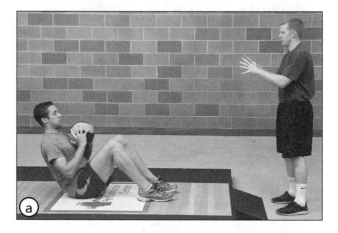

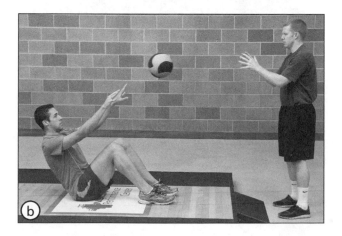

LAT PULLDOWN

Before starting this exercise, the athlete should adjust the seat and the knee pad of the lat machine to fit his body size. The athlete then chooses a comfortable weight. The athlete grips the bar with the hands positioned slightly wider than shoulder width (photo *a*). He sits on the seat and places the knees under the knee pad for support.

1. The athlete leans back slightly at the hips and pulls the bar down to the upper portion of the chest (photo *b*).
2. In a controlled manner, the athlete allows the arms to extend and return to the starting position.

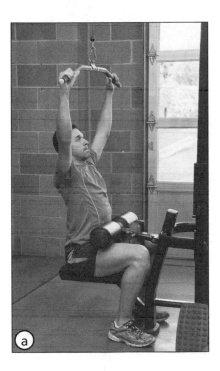
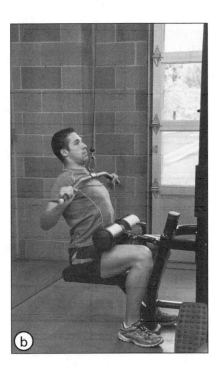

BENT-OVER ROW

The athlete grasps the bar with a closed, pronated grip. The grip should be wider than shoulder width. The athlete positions the feet in a shoulder-width stance with the knees slightly flexed. He flexes the torso forward so that it is slightly above parallel to the floor (photo *a*). Athletes with shorter posterior chain muscles often use a position with cervical extension as shown. Other athletes should use a neutral position for the cervical spine. For the former position, the eyes should be focused ahead, and for the latter, the eyes should be focused a short distance ahead of the feet. The elbows are fully extended so that the bar is hanging down.

1. The athlete pulls the bar toward the torso (photo *b*). He keeps the torso rigid, the back flat, and the knees slightly flexed. The athlete should not jerk the torso upward.
2. The athlete touches the bar to the lower chest or upper abdomen.
3. The athlete lowers the bar back to the starting position while maintaining the flat-back position and keeping the torso and knees stationary.
4. At the end of the set, the athlete flexes the hips and knees to place the bar on the floor and then stands up.

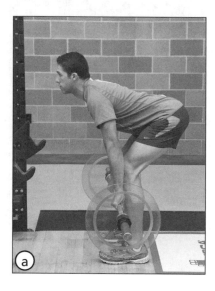 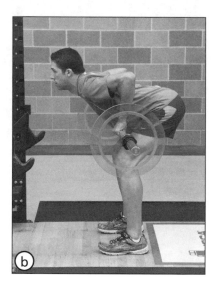

CHIN-UP

The athlete hangs from a bar using an underhand grip with the hands slightly wider than shoulder-width apart (photo *a*). The arms are fully extended.

1. The athlete pulls the body upward until the chin passes above the bar (photo *b*).
2. The athlete then lowers the body back down to the starting position.

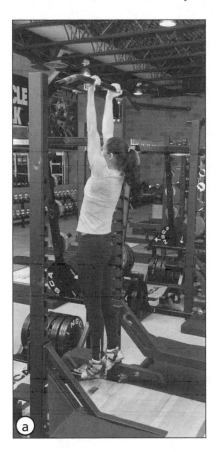 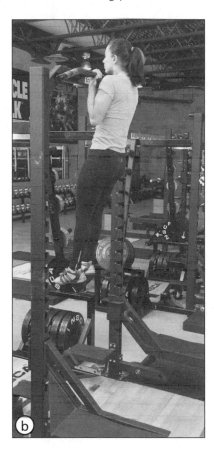

PULL-UP

The athlete hangs from a bar using an overhand grip with the hands slightly wider than shoulder-width apart (photo a). The arms are fully extended.

1. The athlete pulls the body upward until the chin passes above the bar (photo b).
2. The athlete then lowers the body back down to the starting position.

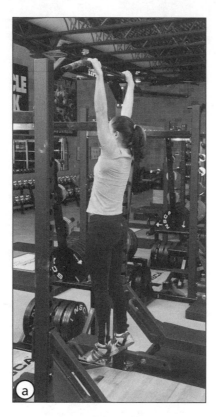 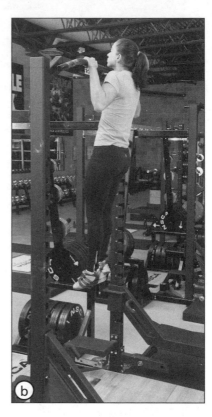

UPRIGHT ROW

The athlete grasps the bar with a closed, pronated grip. The hands should be placed narrower than shoulder-width apart, but no closer than a position where the tips of the thumbs are touching when extended on the bar. The athlete stands erect with the feet shoulder-width apart and the knees slightly flexed. She rests the bar on the front of the thighs (photo *a*); the elbows are fully extended and pointing out to the sides.

1. The athlete pulls the bar up along the abdomen and chest toward the chin. She keeps the elbows pointed out to the sides as she pulls the bar upward. The torso and knees should remain in the same position. The athlete should not rise up on the toes or swing the bar upward.

2. As the athlete moves the bar to the highest position, the elbows move higher than the shoulders and wrists (photo *b*).

3. The athlete allows the bar to slowly descend back to the starting position. She keeps the torso and knees in the same position.

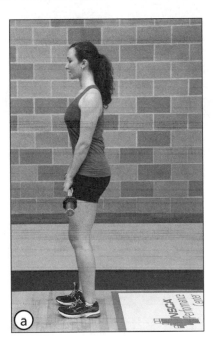 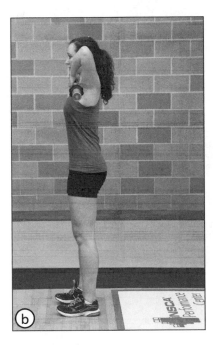

CLEAN-GRIP SHRUG

The athlete grasps the bar using a closed, pronated, clean-width grip (photo *a*). He places the feet shoulder- or hip-width apart with the knees slightly flexed. The torso is erect, the shoulders are held back, and the eyes are focused ahead.

1. The athlete elevates the shoulders straight up as high as possible (trying to touch the shoulders to the ear; photo *b*). The elbows should remain straight.
2. The athlete slowly lowers the bar back down to the starting position.

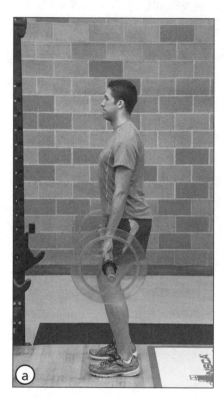
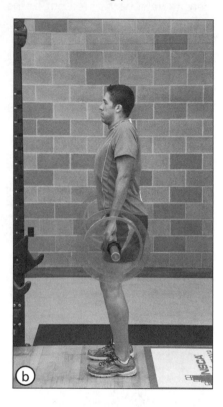

SNATCH-GRIP BEHIND-THE-NECK PRESS

The athlete stands with the feet shoulder-width apart and the knees slightly bent. He maintains a tight torso. Using a snatch grip, the athlete holds the barbell on the back of the shoulders and the middle of the trapezius (photo *a*).

1. The athlete pushes the barbell directly overhead until the elbows are locked out (photo *b*). He pauses with the arms fully extended, maintaining a rigid torso position and a slight bend in the knees and hips.
2. The athlete allows the elbows to slowly flex, lowering the bar to the shoulders and trapezius. He uses the knees as shock absorbers when catching the bar.

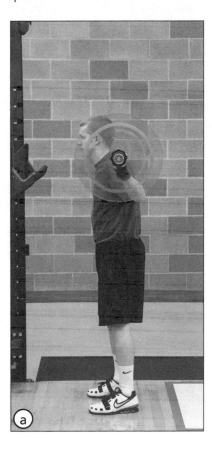
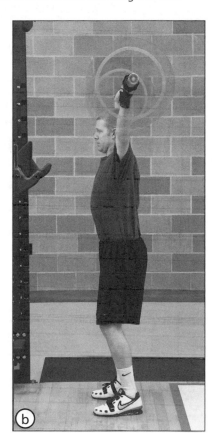

FRONT SHOULDER RAISE

The athlete grasps two dumbbells (or a barbell) using a closed grip. She places the feet shoulder- or hip-width apart with the knees slightly flexed. The torso is erect, the shoulders are held back, and the eyes are focused ahead. The athlete moves the dumbbells to the front of the thighs and positions them with the palms facing the thighs (this creates a pronated grip position; see photo a). The elbows should be slightly flexed throughout the exercise.

1. The athlete begins the exercise by raising the dumbbells up directly in front of the body (photo b). No movement should occur at the elbow joints; movement should occur only at the shoulders. The athlete should not use momentum to assist in performing the movement.

2. The athlete lowers the dumbbells slowly and under control to the starting position.

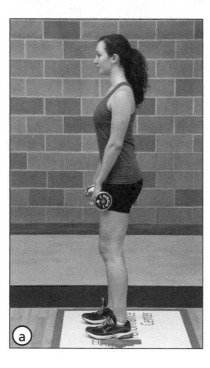 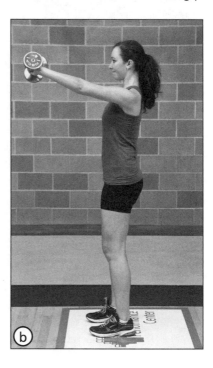

TRICEPS PUSH-DOWN (MACHINE)

The athlete grasps the bar using a closed, pronated grip with the hands 6 to 12 inches (15 to 30 cm) apart. She stands erect with the feet shoulder-width apart and the knees slightly flexed. The athlete positions the body close enough to the machine so the cable hangs straight down. She pulls the bar down to position the upper arms against the sides of the torso (photo a). She flexes the elbows to position the forearms parallel to the floor or slightly above. This is the starting position.

1. The athlete pushes the bar down until the elbows are fully extended (photo b). She keeps the torso erect and the upper arms stationary. The athlete should not forcefully lock out the elbows.

2. The athlete allows the elbows to slowly flex back to the starting position. The torso, upper arms, and knees remain in the same position. At the end of the set, the athlete returns the bar to its resting position.

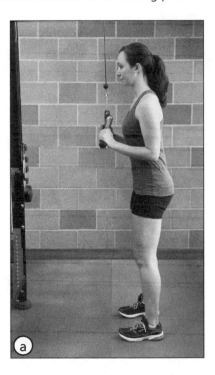 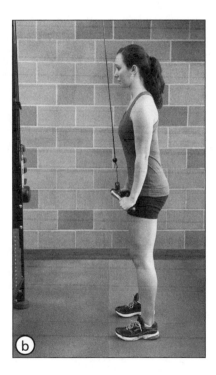

DUMBBELL BICEPS CURL

The athlete grasps two dumbbells using a closed, neutral grip while standing erect with the feet shoulder-width apart and the knees slightly flexed. She positions the dumbbells alongside the thighs with the elbows fully extended (photo *a*). Repetitions begin from this position.

1. Keeping the dumbbell in a neutral grip, the athlete flexes the elbows until the dumbbells clear the thighs on each side; she then supinates the forearms and wrists by turning the hands outward until they are near the anterior deltoids (photo *b*). The athlete keeps the torso erect and the upper arm stationary. She should not jerk the body or swing the dumbbell upward. (The curls can also be performed by alternating arms. The resting arm stays stationary at the side of the thigh.)

2. The athlete lowers the dumbbells until the elbows are fully extended and pronated, moving them back to the neutral starting position.

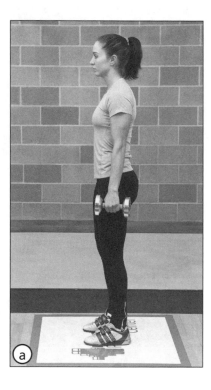 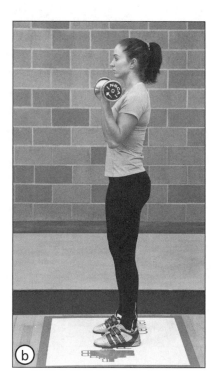

DIP (DIP BAR)

The athlete grasps the handles of the dip bar and assumes an upright position, keeping the elbows straight and using the arms to support his body weight (photo *a*). The knees are bent, and the feet are off the ground.

1. The athlete lowers the body by allowing the elbows to bend until the upper arms are about parallel to the floor or dip bar (photo *b*). He should maintain an erect torso and should not swing the body.

2. The athlete extends the elbows to lift himself back up until the arms are straight (not locked out).

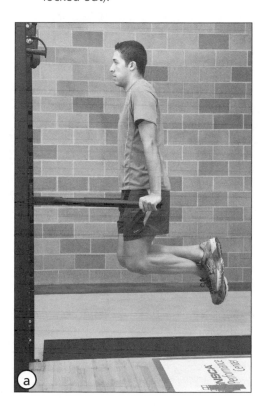
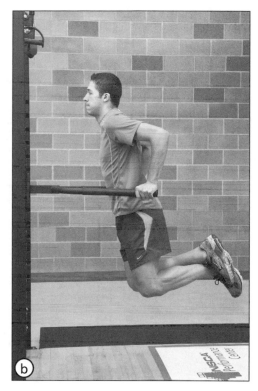

CHAPTER 7

Resistance Training for Endurance Sports

Greg Haff
Stephanie Burgess

Traditionally, endurance athletes have been reluctant to use resistance training as part of their overall training plan. This reluctance has stemmed from the belief that resistance training will result in substantial hypertrophy and weight gain, which would negatively affect performance. Recent scientific evidence appears to refute this belief and offers a compelling argument that resistance training is essential to the overall development of the endurance athlete.

The role that resistance training plays in the development of endurance athletes is a topic that causes a lot of confusion. This chapter offers practical information about the implementation of resistance training programs for endurance athletes based on the current research about concurrent resistance and endurance training. A fundamental part of this discussion is the integration of resistance training into the endurance athlete's training plan.

The process of integrating training factors involves the concept of periodization. Although basic periodization concepts are used by endurance athletes and coaches, these concepts are much more developed and scientifically studied in the application of resistance training. Additionally, the overall depth of planning is substantially greater and the terminology used is slightly different when discussing resistance training. To help endurance coaches develop integrated training programs, this chapter provides a detailed discussion about periodization and how resistance training is built into the overall training plan. From this discussion, practical guidelines are established and presented for the development of effective resistance training programs for the endurance athlete. Finally, sample programs are presented for a variety of endurance sports or activities.

RESISTANCE TRAINING'S EFFECT ON ENDURANCE PERFORMANCE

Endurance athletes who are stronger can generally perform at a much higher level. This suggests that training modalities that stimulate increases in muscular strength without compromising endurance capacity may be beneficial for the endurance athlete. Support for this contention can be found in the scientific literature; research shows that the appropriate integration of resistance training into the endurance athlete's training plan can result in significantly better performance when compared to classic endurance training plans that focus only on aerobic endurance training.

When looking closely at endurance performance, several key factors—including the athlete's maximal aerobic power ($\dot{V}O_2$max), lactate threshold, and movement efficiency—contribute to performance (see figure 7.1). The training modality selected influences these factors by inducing changes to the athlete's aerobic power and capacity, anaerobic capabilities, and neuromuscular function.

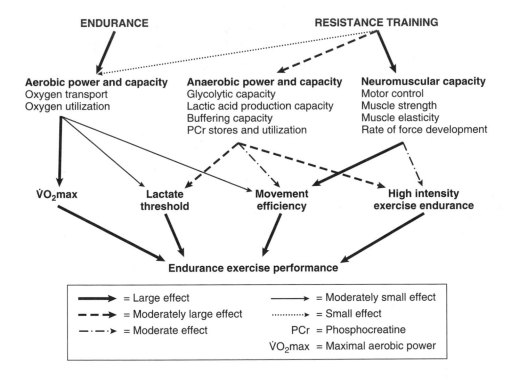

Figure 7.1 The influence of endurance and resistance training on endurance performance.

Adapted, by permission, from L. Paavolainen., K. Häkkinen, I. Hämäläinen, A. Nummela, and H. Rusko, 1999, "Explosive-strength training improves 5-km running time by improving running economy and muscle power," *Journal of Applied Physiology* 86(5): 1527-1533.

Aerobic training exerts a strong influence on both aerobic power and capacity, but it does not exert a great impact on the athlete's anaerobic or neuromuscular abilities. Conversely, resistance training exerts a strong influence on the athlete's neuromuscular function and a moderate influence on anaerobic power and capacity, while offering only a minimal influence on aerobic power and capacity. By influencing the athlete's anaerobic abilities as well as neuromuscular function, resistance training can elevate the athlete's lactate threshold, movement efficiency, and ability to engage in high-intensity activities.

The ability of resistance training to improve endurance performance is likely related to several key factors, including the specific physiological and mechanical adaptations that are stimulated by the resistance training regimen. The integration of resistance training into the overall training plan appears to be central to creating these specific performance-enhancing adaptations.

Traditionally, endurance athletes and coaches have believed that resistance training either does not affect or negatively affects endurance performance. However, this view may be partially explained by a design flaw in many of the training programs that include both resistance and endurance training. The flaw is that resistance training is simply added to the endurance training plan. Athletes who undertake this approach often experience excessively high levels of fatigue that can negatively affect overall performance.

If athletes reduce their endurance training load to account for the addition of resistance training, then resistance training has a positive effect on the athletes' endurance performance. The athlete who performs both resistance and endurance training in an integrated and appropriately planned fashion will perform at a higher level than the athlete who performs only classic endurance training.

MODES AND METHODS OF RESISTANCE TRAINING FOR ENDURANCE

Resistance training is an activity in which the body's skeletal muscle system is required to produce force to overcome some external resistance. This resistance can come from a multitude of devices, including free weights, gravity, resistance machines, and weighted objects. If the resistance applied to the body is planned correctly, with progressive overload, the skeletal muscle system will adapt and become more efficient at generating forces.

A key to the effectiveness of resistance training is the ability to structure training plans that integrate all training factors and appropriately manage total workloads. If the resistance training portion of the training plan is appropriately structured, specific physiological adaptations can occur that result in quantifiable performance improvements. For example, by increasing muscular strength, the endurance runner generally shows improved running economy that translates into improved performance (as indicated by faster times). The extent to which the adaptations induced by resistance training will translate to specific performance outcomes is largely dependent on the mode (type of equipment) and methods (repetitions, sets, volumes, types of movements) used to construct the training plan.

Modes of Resistance Training

Endurance athletes can use numerous modes of resistance training. These modes can include resistance training (exercise) bands or tubing, medicine balls, core stability or balance training (using a stability ball), weight machines, free weights (barbells, dumbbells, kettle balls, weighted vests), plyometrics, and body weight exercises such as push-ups and chin-ups. Depending on the training status of the athlete, each of these modes may have a place in the training plan.

Generally, a combination of free weights, weight machines, body weight exercises, and plyometrics results in the greatest improvements in endurance performance. Conversely, training on unstable surfaces or performing core stability exercises has resulted in no improvements in endurance performance and generally mutes the ability to develop force rapidly. Total-body resistance training, such as squatting, results in a greater activation of the core muscles (lower back and abdominal muscles) when directly compared to core stability exercise. Some modes—such as resistance bands, stability training, and balance training—may be better suited for rehabilitation from injury and should not serve as the focus of any resistance training plan for endurance athletes. Because most training plans for endurance athletes must balance multiple training factors, the best strategy is to employ activities that are time efficient and have the greatest transfer of training effects; this would include modes such as free weights, weight machines, plyometrics, and medicine balls.

Methods of Resistance Training

The methods of resistance training are directly related to the way that the training program is designed. The methods used in the application of resistive loads are largely dictated by the overall goals of the training program or the phase of the periodized training plan. The most effective and time-efficient method for developing strength and power that directly affect athletic performance involves combining several modes of training, such as free weights, plyometrics, and medicine ball work.

Regardless of the mode used, the training plan must progressively overload the athlete. Progressive overload is accomplished through the manipulation of various training factors, such as varying the frequency of training, the volume load (sets × repetitions × load), the intensity of the exercise or session, the rest interval between sets or repetitions, and the exercises used. Too often coaches and sport scientists falsely consider only the variation of volume and intensity of resistance training when attempting to progressively overload the athletes. However, other factors, such as the exercises selected and the order of training, can also significantly influence the effectiveness of the training plan.

Volume

In its most simplistic form, the volume of resistance training is the amount of work accomplished. The best method for estimating the amount of work accomplished in a resistance training session is the calculation of the volume load (sets × repetitions × load). The volume load is a far superior method for estimating the amount of work accomplished because it includes the load in the calculation. If the load is not included in the calculation (sets × repetitions), the result will provide a false representation of volume.

For example, table 7.1 presents four exercises in which the athlete has performed 30 repetitions, which could falsely be interpreted as an equal volume of training. Looking at the volume load calculation, it is clear that the volume of training can differ greatly in response to the load that is lifted. Volume is a representation of work accomplished, so the load should be included in the volume calculation because the load will affect the amount of work undertaken.

Table 7.1   Comparison of Volume Load Calculations

Exercise	Sets	Repetitions	% of 1RM*	Load (kg)	Total repetitions	Volume load (kg)
Back squat	3	10	65%	146.0	30	4,380
Back squat	3	10	55%	124.0	30	3,720
Back squat	2	15	50%	112.5	30	3,375
Back squat	1	30	25%	45.0	30	1,350

*RM = repetition maximum; % of 1RM based off of a maximum back squat of 225 kg.

High volume loads generally result in greater caloric expenditure and can stimulate increases in endurance. Because of this, many endurance athletes believe that they should always perform high-repetition resistance training, which may not be beneficial during certain times in the training year. Periods of high volume load can result in substantial amounts of accumulated fatigue. When high volume loads are encountered too frequently, an endurance athlete may experience a decrease in performance as a result of the fatigue that this type of training stimulates. Endurance athletes must consider the relationship between fatigue, performance, and the volume load of training when integrating a resistance training program into their preparation activities.

Intensity

The intensity of an exercise depends on the rate at which energy is used. Intensity is typically calculated as a percentage of a specified repetition maximum (RM). For example, in table 7.1, three sets of 10 back squats were performed at an intensity of 65 percent (146 kg) of the heaviest weight that could be lifted 1 time, or 1RM, which in this case was 225 kilograms. Working from the initial 1RM is the preferred method of establishing training intensity, but this method does have some potential pitfalls. As the athlete gets stronger, the 1RM increases, and if testing is not undertaken frequently, the training zones become progressively less effective.

One solution for this issue is to work off of goal 1RM values as shown in table 7.2. However, when using this method, the goal established must be realistic so that the athlete does not overtrain. An additional consideration is that the number of repetitions that an athlete can perform at a specific percentage of 1RM varies depending on the exercise and the training experience of the athlete.

Table 7.2 Sample Loading Table

Loading	Intensity	Percentage	% initial 1RM*	% goal 1RM*
Very heavy	(VH)	95-100	213.8-225.0	223.3-235.0
Heavy	(H)	90-95	202.5-213.8	211.5-223.3
Moderately heavy	(MH)	85-90	191.3-202.5	199.8-211.5
Moderate	(M)	80-85	180.0-191.3	188.0-199.8
Moderately light	(ML)	75-80	168.8-180.0	176.3-188.0
Light	(L)	70-75	157.5-168.8	164.5-176.3
Very light	(VL)	<70	<157.5	<164.5

*Goal for an athlete who wants to perform the back squat for 235 kg, who currently can back squat 225 kg for a 1RM.

Adapted from Bompa and Haff, 2009.

Another method is to work from the number of repetitions that can be performed based on percentages of the 1RM, as shown in table 7.3. For example, if an athlete's 1RM is 225 kilograms, his estimated 5RM is approximately 191 kilograms, and his predicted 10RM is around 168 kilograms. Training zones can then be established based on these numbers, as shown in table 7.4. In other words, athletes find their 1RM and then use table 7.3 and the intensity spectrum presented in tables 7.2 and 7.4 to individualize training intensities. This eliminates the need for frequent testing and allows the coach or athlete to use percentages of actual, estimated, or goal RMs.

Table 7.3 Load-to-Repetition Relationship

% of 1RM	Number of repetitions
100	1
95	2
90	3
85	5
80	8
75	10
70	12
65	15

Table 7.4 Sample Loading Ranges Based on Estimated 5RM and 10RM

Loading	Intensity	%	5RM zones*	10RM zones*
Very heavy	(VH)	95-100	182-191	160-168
Heavy	(H)	90-95	172-182	151-160
Moderately heavy	(MH)	85-90	162-172	143-151
Moderate	(M)	80-85	153-162	134-143
Moderately light	(ML)	75-80	143-153	126-134
Light	(L)	70-75	134-143	118-126
Very light	(VL)	<70	<134	<118

*Athlete has a 1RM back squat of 225 kg; therefore, based on table 7.3, the athlete's estimated 5RM is 191 kg and his 10RM is 168 kg.

Adapted from Bompa and Haff, 2009.

Repetitions

The number of repetitions that an athlete can perform is determined by the load. The higher the load used, the lower the number of repetitions that can be performed, and vice versa. Many factors may contribute to the number of repetitions that an athlete can perform at a given percentage of 1RM. Table 7.3 offers a rough guideline that can be used when creating a training plan.

One concept that must be considered is that the repetition scheme employed can result in specific physiological adaptations. As depicted in figure 7.2, repetition schemes of over 20 repetitions can enhance low-intensity endurance, while those

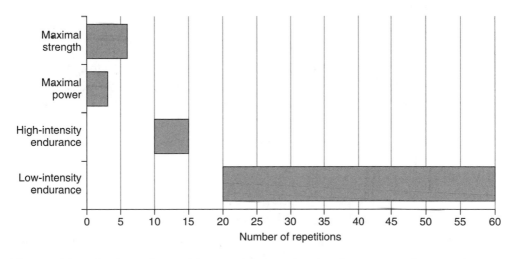

Figure 7.2 Number of repetitions needed to develop four types of strength.

Adapted, by permission, from T.O. Bompa and G.G. Haff, 2009, *Periodization: Theory and methodology of training*, 5th ed. (Champaign, IL: Human Kinetics) 274.

of 10 to 15 repetitions can enhance high-intensity endurance. Overall maximal strength is best developed with repetition schemes that range from 1 to 6 repetitions, and power is developed with lower-repetition models of 3 or fewer repetitions. The selection of the repetition range should be based on the goals established for the phases of the training plan as well as the physiological adaptations targeted.

Sets

Sets are a series of repetitions performed continuously followed by a rest interval. Multiple-set protocols are significantly more effective than single-set programs because they stimulate greater physiological adaptations and result in greater performance gains. The number of sets used in a training program is largely dependent on the training status of the athlete, the phase of training, and the targeted goals of the training plan.

Advanced athletes generally need to perform a greater number of sets (more than three) per exercise, while novice athletes can achieve performance gains with fewer sets (three or fewer). Manipulating the number of sets is another method for modifying the volume load of training. Increasing the number of sets increases volume load, while decreasing the number of sets reduces the volume load.

Variation in the number of sets used in the resistance training program will be dictated by the phase of training. For example, early in the training year, during the preparatory phase, the number of sets would be greater in order to increase the overall volume load and to develop muscular endurance. Conversely, during the competitive phase, a lower number of sets will be used because of the reduced emphasis on resistance training.

Rest Interval Between Sets

The time allotted between sets, or the rest interval, is a function of the load being lifted, the goal of the training program, and the type of strength being targeted. When targeting the development of muscular strength or power, a long rest interval of 2 to 5 minutes may be warranted. Conversely, when attempting to develop muscular endurance, shortening the rest interval to less than 2 minutes may be advantageous. Programs with short rest intervals will likely result in specific physiological adaptations that can facilitate the performance of endurance-based activities.

Order of Exercises

As a general rule, multijoint exercises that involve a large muscle mass, such as the back squat or power clean, should be performed early in the training session. These types of exercises are often technical and require the athlete to be in a state of minimal fatigue in order to maximize their effectiveness. These exercises should be considered the most important exercises in the resistance training program.

Exercises that involve a smaller muscle mass, such as biceps curls or triceps push-downs, are generally performed after the large-mass exercises have been completed. If an athlete chooses to perform the smaller-mass exercises first, this may reduce the effectiveness of the multijoint exercises. For example, if the athlete chooses to perform a triceps exercise (triceps are an accessory muscle for shoulder press exercises) before the bench press, then fatigue of the triceps would likely prevent the ability to overload the anterior deltoid and pectoralis major.

Training Frequency

Training frequency refers to the number of resistance training sessions that will be undertaken during the training plan. As a general rule, the endurance athlete needs no more than three resistance training sessions per week. In fact, endurance athletes will likely perform a maximum of two resistance training sessions per week during most of the annual training plan.

Because resistance training is a supplemental training activity for the endurance athlete, less emphasis is placed on this type of training; thus, fewer sessions per week are warranted. The frequency of resistance training for these athletes may be as high as 3 days per week during the preparatory phase and as low as 1 day per week during the competitive phase of the annual training plan. Additionally, resistance training may be completely removed from the training plan during the pre-event taper in order to maximize the removal of accumulated fatigue.

Loading Pattern

Normally, the loading pattern should contain a series of warm-up sets followed by target sets in which a prescribed repetition and intensity scheme is followed. For example, if an athlete were to perform target sets in the back squat at 70 kilograms (50 percent of 1RM) for 3 sets of 10, the athlete would do 2 or 3 warm-up sets before initiating the target sets. The warm-up sets may be structured as follows: 1 set at 20 kilograms, 1 set at 40 kilograms, and 1 set at 60 kilograms. After completing the warm-up sets, the athlete would perform the target sets. In some instances, a down set may be used as a cool-down. In the example, the athlete might perform a down set with 52.5 kilograms (or a 25 percent reduction in load).

Another consideration for the loading pattern involves manipulating the intensity and volume load throughout the training week (see table 7.5 on page 106). As a general rule, the intensity of training should not be the same every day and should be integrated with the endurance training plan. The table depicts a 3:1 loading program. In a 3:1 loading program, intensity (and volume load) increases for 3 consecutive weeks, followed by 1 week of unloading, which is used to induce recovery. Within each week, the training load decreases with each training day as fatigue accumulates during the week.

Table 7.5 Sample Loading Pattern for a Training Week

Day	Target zone		Intensities*			
	Sets	Reps	Week 1	Week 2	Week 3	Week 4
Loading pattern for a 3-day-a-week program						
Monday	3	10	ML	M	MH	M
Wednesday	3	10	L	ML	M	ML
Friday	3	10	VL	L	ML	L
Loading pattern for a 2-day-a-week program						
Tuesday	3	10	ML	M	MH	M
Friday	3	10	L	ML	M	ML

*Intensities based on table 7.4.

Because most endurance athletes perform the greatest volume of endurance work on the weekend, these athletes may want to reverse this loading program so that the light day is at the beginning of the week. This way, the program addresses the fatigue created in response to the higher volumes of endurance training undertaken during the weekend. Ultimately, the major factor that will dictate this manipulation of the resistance training load will be how the endurance training is sequenced and integrated into the overall training plan.

STRUCTURE AND SEQUENCE OF ENDURANCE RESISTANCE TRAINING

Once an athlete has decided to use resistance training to improve endurance performance, the athlete and coach must then determine the overall goals of the athlete, the specific needs of the athlete, and the target of the training plan. After establishing the athlete's overall goals, the coach and athlete can work together to craft a training program that effectively integrates training factors in order to facilitate the athlete's progress.

One of the keys to designing an appropriate resistance training program for endurance athletes is the concept of periodization. Periodization can be defined as the logical and systematic sequencing and integration of training factors in order to optimize performance at specific times. Periodization should be considered a planning process.

Central to this concept is the fact that not every training factor needs to be emphasized at the same time. In fact, as the athlete moves through the training year, the focus of the training plan should shift, allowing training factors to be introduced, removed, or reintroduced at predetermined points. Thus, for the endurance athlete who has integrated resistance training into a periodized training plan, the plan will include specific time frames for targeting the development of strength, power, or muscular endurance. For these factors to be integrated at the appropriate time, the training plan must be broken into specific training periods and phases, which serve as the foundation of the overall training plan.

From a structural standpoint, a training plan can be broken into the five units or periods shown in table 7.6. The largest period is the multiyear plan, which is usually designed based on a four-year structure. The multiyear plan provides a general overview of what the athlete is attempting to accomplish in the long term. For example, in a high school setting, the program focus of a freshman cross country runner will differ greatly from that of a senior who has been engaged in directed training for three consecutive annual training plans or macrocycles (see figure 7.3 on page 158). The foundation of each macrocycle is the competitive schedule, which is used to establish the phases that will be included in the annual training plan.

Table 7.6   Defining Specific Training Periods

Period	Duration	Description
Multiyear plan	2 to 4 years	Also called a quadrennial plan
Macrocycle	Several months to a year	Sometimes referred to as an annual plan Contains a preparatory, competitive, and transition phase of training
Mesocycle	2 to 6 weeks	Medium-sized training cycle Sometimes referred to as a macrocycle or a block of training Consists of microcycles that are linked together
Microcycle	Several days to 2 weeks	Small training cycle composed of multiple workouts
Workout	Several hours	Generally consists of several hours of training More than 30 minutes of rest between bouts would constitute multiple workouts

Sources: Issurin 2008a; Issurin 2008b, p. 213; Stone, Stone, and Sands 2007, p. 376; Siff 2003, p. 496; Bompa and Haff 2009.

Macrocycles

The multiyear plan serves as the template that is used to establish the individual annual training plans, or macrocycles. Generally, the macrocycle will be a year in duration, but depending on the sport, a macrocycle could be structured to last several months. For example, an endurance athlete at the high school level may have a fall cross country season and a spring track season. In this scenario, two macrocycles would be designed to address the needs of each season. Regardless of the number of macrocycles, the basic structure contains specific training and performance goals that are sequenced in the context of the multiyear plan.

So in our example of the cross country runner in a high school setting, the macrocycle for the freshman will be designed with specific goals for establishing a performance foundation; these goals may place a major emphasis on the development of cardiovascular fitness and muscular strength, while deemphasizing the importance of competitive performances. With each successive macrocycle, the athlete will continue to develop these physiological and performance characteristics, but the focus on competitive performances will increase. In the fourth year of the multiyear plan, the macrocycle will be designed to result in an optimization of performance, allowing the athlete to achieve his greatest performance times or competitive success.

Generally, the macrocycle is broken into three major phases—preparatory, competitive, and transition (see table 7.7). The preparatory phase is the first phase of every macrocycle. This phase can vary in length depending on the developmental level of the athlete, the requirements of the sport, the length of the macrocycle, and the amount of time before the major competitions. The major focus of this phase is the development of the athlete's overall physical capacity through the use of higher-volume training, which is performed with lower intensities.

The preparatory phase can be subdivided into the general preparatory and specific preparatory phases. The general preparatory subphase occurs first and is used to emphasize basic skills, increase working capacity, and elevate overall physical preparation. In the case of resistance training, this subphase generally targets the development of strength endurance. In the specific preparatory subphase, the training emphasis will shift toward the incorporation of more sport-specific conditioning activities while continuing to increase the athlete's working capacity. In the case of resistance training, a shift from strength endurance to the development of basic strength will occur as the athlete transitions into the specific preparatory phase. As the athlete progresses through this subphase, performance levels should rise as the athlete becomes prepared for the competitive phase of the macrocycle.

The second major phase of the macrocycle is the competitive phase. The duration of the competitive phase is largely dependent on the competition schedule and the relative importance of these competitions. Ultimately, the competitive phase should target a specific major competition in which the athlete's performance will be maximized. As the athlete moves through the competitive phase, the training activities become more specific, and the emphasis on performance becomes greater.

The competitive phase is subdivided into the precompetitive and main competitive subphases. The precompetitive subphase includes activities used to maintain sport-specific fitness while elevating the athlete's level of performance. Additionally, minor competitions or exhibitions are used to evaluate the athlete's progress toward the targeted goals established for the main competitive subphase. The main competitive subphase includes the major competitions in which the athlete's performance is expected to be maximized. The maximization of performance is accomplished through the manipulation of training variables to help the athlete maintain sport-specific fitness while decreasing the overall level of fatigue. From a

Table 7.7 Phases of the Annual Training Plan

Phase	Characteristics	
Preparatory	• Contains an overall high volume of training with a lower intensity • Designed to increase overall physical capacity • Cultivates specific psychological traits • Familiarizes the athlete with the basic technical and tactical aspects of the sport	
	Subphases	
	General preparatory	• Primary emphasis on basic skills with a lesser emphasis on sport-specific skills • Increases the athlete's working capacity • Elevates overall physical preparation • Improves basic technical elements • Enhances basic tactical abilities • High overall volume of training
	Specific preparatory	• Emphasis of training shifts from basic skills to sport-specific skills • Increases the athlete's working capacity • Greater emphasis on specialized skills and technical elements related to the sport • Elevates overall athletic performance
Competitive	• Incorporates competitions of varying levels of importance • Targets the improvement of sport-specific physical attributes • Maximizes performance level • Perfects technical and tactical skills • Maintains sport-specific fitness • Diminishes fatigue and elevates preparedness	
	Subphases	
	Precompetitive	• Includes unofficial or minor competitions designed to evaluate the athlete's preparedness • Maintains sport-specific fitness • Increases performance level • Includes decreases in volume along with increases in intensity of training
	Main competitive	• Includes gradual decreases in training volume in order to reduce fatigue and elevate performance • Designed to maximize performance and peak the athlete at specific times • Contains specific peaking strategies that include modulating the volume and intensity of training
Transition	• Serves as a link between macrocycles • Prepares the athlete for the next macrocycle of training • Is used to induce recovery from training stress and injuries • Includes training at a substantially reduced level in order to maintain some general fitness • Generally lasts between 2 and 6 weeks	

Adapted from Bompa and Haff, 2009.

resistance training standpoint, the precompetitive and main competitive subphases generally contain training activities that are designed to emphasize the development of strength and power.

After the completion of the competitive phase, athletes usually move into a transition or active rest phase of training. This phase serves as a link between macrocycles and is designed to induce recovery from the competitive season. In some cases, this is also a time for the athlete to heal from any injuries that may have occurred during the season. This phase is marked by substantially reduced training levels. However, the athlete must be sure to undertake some training activities during this phase in order to maintain or slow the loss of general fitness. Depending on the needs of the athlete and the time allotted, the transition phase will last between 2 and 6 weeks. The transition phase is an essential portion of the macrocycle and must be established when constructing the overall annual training plan.

Mesocycles, Microcycles, and Workouts

Once the macrocycle phases and subphases are established, smaller training units, known as mesocycles, can be designed. Mesocycles consist of 2- to 6-week periods of training that target specific physiological and performance objectives based on the goals established for the specific phases (i.e., general preparatory, specific preparatory, precompetitive, and competitive phase) of the macrocycle. Depending on the goals established for the macrocycle, various mesocycle structures can be developed (see table 7.8). Each mesocycle contained within the macrocycle should be interlinked or sequenced so that each mesocycle builds on the adaptations established in the previous mesocycle.

For example, in the general preparatory phase, the mesocycle plan for resistance training will focus on the development of muscular endurance, which would be accomplished by performing higher-repetition, lower-intensity training. Conversely, during the competitive phase, the goal for the mesocycle is to elevate performance; for endurance athletes, resistance training may now target high-power movements and the reduction of accumulated fatigue. The mesocycle plan would address the development of fatigue by including a significant decrease in overall training loads 8 to 14 days before the major competition (e.g., the state championships in high school track and field). This reduction allows for a reduction in fatigue and an elevation in performance.

Each individual week within the mesocycle is referred to as a microcycle. For the endurance athlete, the structure of a microcycle will depend on the location of the microcycle within the larger planning structures (i.e., mesocycle, macrocycle, and annual training plan), the individual athlete's needs, and the time available for structured training. The microcycle is generally 7 days in duration; however,

Table 7.8 Sample Mesocycle Structures

Type	Average duration (weeks)	Characteristics
Basic sport specific	6	• Designed to elevate sport-specific fitness where performance in specific skills is targeted
Buildup	3	• A more general form of training and conditioning that is used to enhance foundational skills or fitness • May be used after a period of specific or high-load training
Competition	2-6	• A mesocycle that specifically targets a competition during that mesocycle • Used in the competitive phase of the annual training plan
Competitive buildup	3	• A period of increasing training loads that occurs during a long competitive phase • Used to reestablish foundational skills or fitness
General	Any duration	• Basic or general education and training that target the development of basic fitness • Often occurs in the preparatory phase of the annual training plan
Immediate preparatory	2	• A training period that occurs before a competition • Targets peaking and recovery • May be considered a taper • May precede a testing period
Precompetitive	6	• A training period used to maximize preparedness and performance for a specific competition or series of competitions • Marked by sport-specific training • Designed to peak fitness, performance, and preparedness
Preparatory	6	• Designed to develop a base necessary for competitive performance • Training moves from extensive to intensive • Fitness is established and used to develop skills
Recovery	1-4	• Has a specific goal of inducing recovery • May occur after a series of competitions • Serves to prepare the athlete for subsequent training
Stabilization	4	• Training used to perfect technique and fitness base • Targets technical errors as well as fitness deficits • Used to develop sport-specific fitness and base of skills

Adapted, by permission, from M.H. Stone, M. Stone, and W.A. Sands, 2007, *Principles and practice of resistance training* (Champaign, IL: Human Kinetics), 9. Also adapted from D. Harre, 1982, *Trainingslehre* (Berlin: Sportverlag).

this is not a steadfast rule. The 7-day microcycle structure is most commonly seen during the preparatory phase—the phase in which no competitions are planned. In the competitive phase, the microcycle will often be less than 7 days. Various types of microcycles can be used to stimulate specific physiological and performance adaptations. In fact, many sport scientists and coaches believe that the microcycle is one of the most important components of the planning process because it is used to structure the individual training days and daily workout schedules.

The microcycle is the foundation from which the contents of each individual training day are developed. Remember that the number of training days within the microcycle is dependent on many factors, including the athlete's level of development, the time available for training, and the overall phase of the meso- and macrocycle. For example, during the preparatory phase for a novice endurance athlete, the microcycle may contain 3 training days that include resistance training and only 3 or 4 days of specific endurance training. Conversely, during the competitive phase, the number of training days that include resistance training could be reduced (fewer than 3 days) or completely removed so that more emphasis can be placed on endurance training. Generally, the more advanced endurance athlete will have more training days within the microcycle, and the novice or recreational athlete will have fewer training days.

The training day can be further divided into individual workouts, the smallest training periods. The length of the workout can vary, but a workout will generally include several hours of focused training. From a structural standpoint, if 30 minutes or more of rest occurs between two bouts of training in the same day, then these bouts are two workouts. Thus, multiple training goals may be targeted within the training day by separating sessions by short periods of rest (30 minutes or more) or by spacing multiple workouts throughout the training day. The number of workouts in a training day will depend on the athlete's level of development, ability to tolerate training stress, and time available for training.

The sequencing of the workout sessions within the microcycle must be considered because the fatigue generated by one session can affect the athlete's ability to perform during the next workout. If the endurance athlete performs two workouts within one training day, the effects of the first workout may result in a reduced training capacity during the second workout. This is particularly evident when minimal recovery time is provided between workouts.

For example, if the endurance athlete performs a heavy resistance training workout followed by an endurance training session, the overall quality of the endurance training session would be significantly reduced (as a result of the fatigue generated by the resistance training workout). If the primary target of the training day is the development of strength, this structure would be appropriate; however, the two workouts must be separated to allow the athlete to recover from the resistance training bout before performing the endurance training session. This may be accomplished by scheduling the resistance training workout in the morning and the endurance workout in the afternoon. Table 7.9 lists options for how to sequence resistance training and endurance workouts within a training day, along with the likely ramifications of each option.

Table 7.9 Options for the Order of Resistance and Endurance Workouts

Option	Time	Training session focus	Comments
1	a.m.	Resistance training	This order places emphasis on the resistance training and requires a lower intensity and volume of training in the PM endurance workout. This order may be best suited for the general preparatory phase.
	p.m.	Endurance training	
2	a.m.	Endurance training	This order places emphasis on the endurance training and requires a lower intensity and volume of training in the PM resistance training session. This order can be used in the specific preparatory or competitive phase.
	p.m.	Resistance training	
3	a.m. or p.m.	Resistance training and endurance training	This order places emphasis on the resistance training. Because the bouts of exercise are performed in close proximity to one another, this order results in a reduced anabolic response being induced by the resistance training. In addition, technical changes resulting from fatigue may occur during the endurance bout.
4	a.m. or p.m.	Endurance training and resistance training	This order places emphasis on the endurance training. Because the bouts of exercise are performed in close proximity to one another, this order results in a magnification of inflammation and greater protein degradation.

SEQUENCING RESISTANCE TRAINING

For any training plan to be effective, the training activities must result in physiological and performance gains that directly translate into improvements in competitive performance. One of the primary factors in achieving this is the sequencing of the various types of training. Four major categories of resistance training exist: strength endurance, basic strength, strength power, and peaking or maintenance. These different goals are achieved by manipulating the training volume, intensity, duration, and number of repetitions or sets.

The development of strength endurance is best suited for the early portion of the preparatory phase and serves as a tool for developing a training base. In this phase, the volume load of training is the highest; thus, a greater reduction in the overall volume and intensity of endurance training is required. Because of this very high volume load of training, the athlete may only be able to target this category for 1 to 4 weeks. Training for strength endurance is generally undertaken before the development of basic strength.

The second category of training that can be included in the preparatory phase is the development of basic strength. This category of resistance training is marked by a reduction in volume load along with a significant increase in training intensity, which is designed to increase the athlete's strength levels. Generally, resistance training that targets the development of basic strength is undertaken for 1 to 4 weeks. Although an emphasis on basic strength development is typically seen in the preparatory phase, this type of training may also be used in the precompetitive phase of a long competitive season. The development of basic strength serves as the foundation that allows power-generating capacity to be elevated.

The development of strength power generally occurs during the competitive phase and is marked by very high intensities and low volumes of training. For this category, the training objectives target the continued elevation of muscular strength while maximizing the athlete's power output. Generally, the athlete can target these attributes for 1 to 4 weeks before having to alter the training focus.

The final resistance training category is either a peaking or a maintenance program. The decision on whether to use a peaking or maintenance program is largely dictated by the sport. If the sport includes a competitive season that requires a high level of performance over a prolonged period of time, the athlete should use a maintenance program. In most instances, however, the endurance athlete will target a specific competition in which performance will be peaked. When the athlete is attempting to peak for one major competition, the training program will include a 40 to 60 percent reduction in training load (volume and intensity) 8 to 14 days before the competition, allowing for the dissipation of accumulated fatigue. The magnitude of the reduction of training load will depend on the length of the taper (period of time before the competition); short tapers (closer to 8 days) will include a greater reduction than longer tapers (closer to 14 days). Ultimately, the reduction in training load will result in a maximization of performance capacity.

The four categories of resistance training should be viewed as a training continuum on which the appropriate sequencing of training is based. Generally, the basic sequencing pattern is as follows:

Strength endurance → Basic strength →
Strength power → Peaking or maintenance

The general sequence can be used in most situations, but it is not set in stone and can be modified as follows when the preparatory phase is long:

Strength endurance → Basic strength → Strength endurance →
Basic strength → Strength power → Peaking or maintenance

Note that the smallest time frame used for training within one of these specific categories is 1 week and that training should not be done for multiple categories simultaneously. The physiological adaptations achieved in each category facilitate the development that occurs in the next category in the training continuum. For example, in order to tolerate the increased training load encountered during the basic strength category, an athlete must first create an appropriate base of strength endurance. Similarly, basic strength must be developed before the athlete can maximize power-generating ability. Attempting to perform training for all categories in one training session or during 1 week of training can result in excessive fatigue and an inability to integrate resistance training with the endurance portion of the training plan.

INTEGRATION OF ENDURANCE RESISTANCE TRAINING

As previously noted, an essential part of adding resistance training to an endurance athlete's training plan is to successfully integrate the two types of training. Simply adding resistance training to an existing endurance training plan causes greater levels of fatigue and an overall increased workload. Endurance athletes in this situation often report more fatigue than normal and an inability to sustain the planned training volumes. Special care must be taken to modulate the training loads of both the resistance and endurance portions of the training plan in order to appropriately manage the accumulated fatigue.

The most important integration strategy is to reduce the amount of endurance training to accommodate the addition of resistance training. No consensus exists in the scientific literature about the exact amount of reduction required to accommodate the addition of resistance training. Studies reporting improved endurance performance from using a combination of endurance and resistance training reduced the amount of endurance training by 19 to 37 percent.

Determining the proper amount of reduction depends on the phase of training, the amount of resistance training included in the program, and the goals of the annual training plan. For example, during the general preparation phase, the endurance athlete should reduce the amount of endurance training by a greater percent (25 to 37 percent) because of the greater frequency and volume of resistance training. During the competitive phase, however, endurance training could be reduced at a lower percentage (19 to 25 percent) because of the lower workload (frequency and volume) of resistance training within this phase.

Regardless of the training phase, athletes and coaches must pay attention to total workload and the collective effects of both endurance and resistance training. They must consider how the two types of training are integrated. Though reducing the frequency of endurance training when adding resistance training seems to make sense, coaches and athletes often view this approach unfavorably. Endurance athletes often believe that they need frequent training sessions—usually 5 or 6 days per week.

The scientific literature seems to support the endurance athlete's desire to maintain this level of frequency. When reducing endurance training loads before a competition (during a taper), the best approach is to decrease the volume and intensity of individual training sessions rather than decrease the frequency of training. Using this practice during a taper results in significantly higher performance levels. This approach also allows the athlete to reduce the overall workload of endurance training to accommodate the addition of resistance training.

Another important consideration for integration relates to the order of the endurance and resistance training (as discussed previously and highlighted in table 7.9 on page 151). When athletes complete resistance training in the morning and endurance training in the afternoon, a reasonable plan would be to complete an easier afternoon workout to accommodate the fatigue from the morning workout. This strategy would be necessary when targeting strength development and may be best suited for the general preparatory subphase. Switching the order of the workouts would negatively affect the resistance training workout. This sequencing may be best suited for the specific preparatory subphase or during portions of the competitive phase of the macrocycle.

Regardless of the order of the workouts, athletes and coaches must consider the effects of each training session when constructing a comprehensive training plan that includes both resistance and endurance training. Athletes should avoid performing high-volume, high-intensity resistance and endurance training on the same day. If the volume and intensity of the resistance training are high, the subsequent endurance session should be a low-volume, low-intensity recovery session. However, if the volume and intensity of the resistance training are low, the endurance session can be of a higher volume and intensity. When integrating resistance training, endurance athletes must ensure that the sessions or workouts are sequenced in the context of the overall workload. Giving careful thought to these factors when designing the training plan will increase the chances of success.

DESIGN OF ENDURANCE RESISTANCE TRAINING

When developing a resistance training plan, endurance athletes and coaches can employ a sequential planning process as shown in table 7.10. The basic process of integrating resistance training into the endurance athlete's plan should begin with defining the objectives for the training plan. After establishing the objectives, the coach or athlete will then define the macrocycle structure, outline the basic structure of the mesocycles, construct the individual microcycle plans, determine the structure of training days, and establish the individual workouts.

Table 7.10 Sequential Planning Process for Resistance Training

Step 1	Determine the target objectives for the annual training plan.
	Planning tasks:
	  1. Identify the target performance goals.
	  2. Determine performance tests or standards to target during training.
	  3. Define the goals and objectives for the resistance training program.
	  4. Identify the objectives for the endurance training portion of the training plan.

Step 2	Define the macrocycle structure.
	Planning tasks:
	  1. Define the competition schedule.
	  2. Determine when the most important competitions will take place.
	  3. Identify any planned time off (e.g., for student-athletes, identify when classes are not in session).
	  4. Determine when the athlete may be training without a coach.
	  5. Specify when the preparatory and competitive subphases will occur.
	  6. Identify when the general and specific preparatory subphases will be conducted.
	  7. Indicate when the precompetitive and competitive subphases will occur.
	  8. Determine when the transition and recovery phases will occur.
	  9. Establish the specific points when the athlete is planning to peak and indicate this by using the peaking index (see page 157).

Step 3	Outline the basic structure of the mesocycles.
	Planning tasks:
	  1. Determine the emphasis of the training phase.
	  2. Define the length of the mesocycles.
	  3. Integrate the phases and factors targeted in the training plan with the mesocycle structure.
	  4. Indicate when performance tests are to be conducted.

Step 4	Construct the individual microcycle plans.
	Planning tasks:
	  1. Identify the number of resistance training days, endurance training days, and speed training days in each microcycle.
	  2. Indicate the volume of resistance, endurance, and speed training in each microcycle.
	  3. Define the intensity of resistance, endurance, and speed training in each microcycle.
	  4. Determine the duration and distance of the endurance training in each microcycle.
	  5. Indicate when recovery microcycles will take place.

Step 5	Determine the structure of training days.
	Planning tasks:
	  1. Determine the number of training sessions for each training day.
	  2. Define the daily training sequence.
	  3. Identify the intensity and volume of training within each training day.

Step 6	Establish the individual workouts.
	Planning tasks:
	  1. Establish the training goals for each workout.
	  2. Define the warm-up, training, and cool-down activities.
	  3. Order the training activities according to importance and how fatigue will affect the activities.
	  4. Sequence the training activities.

Define the Macrocycle Structure

After establishing the athlete's goals and objectives for the annual training plan, the most crucial step in the planning process is to establish the competitive calendar. One of the best methods for mapping out the competitive calendar is to use an annual training plan template. Using this template, the coach can indicate when each competition is, where the competition is located, and the relative importance of the competition.

For example, when working with a collegiate distance runner who competes in the Big East Conference, we would break the annual training plan into three macrocycles; when combined, these macrocycles run from June to May (see figure 7.3 on page 158). The first macrocycle encompasses the cross country season and culminates in a major peak on November 1st at the Big East Cross Country Championships.

This macrocycle is subdivided into two major phases: the preparatory phase and the competitive phase. The preparatory phase lasts 12 weeks and runs from June until the week ending August 23rd. This phase is subdivided into the general preparatory subphase, which lasts 7 weeks, and the specific preparatory subphase, which lasts 5 weeks. The competitive phase lasts 10 weeks and runs from the end of the preparatory phase until the competition on the week ending November 1st. This phase is subdivided into the precompetitive and competitive subphases. The precompetitive subphase will include some exhibitions or competitions of minor importance that serve as situational practices where performance is not expected to be peaked. Conversely, performance is expected to elevate across the competitive subphase, resulting in a major peak at the Big East Championship at the end of the competitive phase.

After the major competition, the athlete will transition into the second macrocycle. A 2-week transition phase is initiated in which training stress is minimized to allow the athlete to recover from the preceding competitive phase. The second macrocycle lasts 16 weeks (November 1st to February 21st), including the 2-week transition phase, a 10-week preparatory phase, and a 4-week competitive phase. Because the indoor track season is considered of minor importance for this athlete, a longer preparatory phase is used, and the athlete is not brought to a major peak.

Six weeks of the preparatory phase will be dedicated to general preparation, and only 4 weeks will be focused on specific preparatory activities. During the specific preparatory subphase, the athlete participates in two competitions, but they are used as training days. In the competitive phase, the precompetitive subphase is relatively short, lasting only 2 weeks. This subphase results in some elevation in performance, but the athlete does not peak. The competitive subphase is also relatively short (only 2 weeks), but the athlete reaches a minor peak.

The third macrocycle will be initiated without a transition phase, but the first microcycle of the preparatory phase will contain some recovery sessions, especially early in the week. This preparatory phase is relatively short, lasting only 4 weeks; only 2 weeks are dedicated to both the general and specific preparatory subphases. The competitive phase is 6 weeks long with only 2 weeks for the precompetitive subphase. The competitive subphase is 4 weeks in duration and brings the athlete to a major peak. After competing in the Big East Outdoor Track and Field Championships, this athlete would perform a 4-week transition phase before initiating the next annual training plan.

Once the annual training plan is outlined, the individual macrocycles are established, and the phases of training are defined, the coach should identify the important competitions. This is an essential step because it allows the coach to establish when the athlete will be at peak preparedness. To indicate this, coaches often use a tool called the peaking index. The peaking index is a 5-point scale with 5 indicating the lowest level of preparedness and 1 indicating a peak or maximum level of preparedness. As a general rule, the peaking index will be at 4 or 5 during the preparatory phase, because this phase involves a high volume of training that leads to a lot of cumulative fatigue. Conversely, during the competitive phase, the peaking index will be closer to 1; with the lower training volume and appropriate planning, the athlete's level of preparedness will rise as fatigue is dissipated and more emphasis is placed on preparing for competition. Figure 7.3 on page 158 shows the appropriate peaking index to help establish the training objectives for each phase.

Some coaches and athletes think that developing an annual training plan is too time consuming, and they choose to skip this step in the planning process. This is a mistake because a carefully crafted annual training plan allows the coach to better integrate the training factors. Developing the annual plan is of particular importance when resistance training will be included in the endurance athlete's training schedule. The annual training plan can be used to estimate when training stressors will be highest, to determine the targeted peaking times, and to better manage the workloads that the athlete will use in training. After the annual training plan is established, the structure and focus of the mesocycles can be added to the planning chart (see figure 7.3 on page 158).

	Month	June				July				August			
Date	Week	7	14	21	28	5	12	19	26	2	9	16	23
Competition	Domestic												
	International												
	Name of competition												
Periodization	Training phase	Preparatory 1											
	Training subphase	General								Specific			
	Macrocycle	Macrocycle 1											
	Mesocycle	1				2				3			
	Microcycle	1	2	3	4	5	6	7	8	9	10	11	12
	Resistance training	3	3	3	3	3	3	3	3	2	2	2	
	Endurance training	6	6	6	6	6	6	6	6	6	6	6	
	Speed training												
	Peaking index	5	5	5	5	5	5	5	4	4	4	4	4
	Testing dates	▨											
	Recovery weeks				U				U				U
Resistance training	Sets x repetitions	3 x 15	3 x 15	3 x 15	3 x 15	3 x 5	3 x 5	3 x 5	3 x 5	3 x 10	3 x 10	3 x 10	3 x 10
	Intensity	VL	L	ML	L	ML	M	MH	ML	L	ML	M	L
	Strength-endurance												
	Basic strength												
	Strength-power												
	Peaking												
Endurance training	Time												
	Distance												
	Intensity												

Work load (scale 0–100)

Symbols		Peaking index	Abbreviations
■	Major peak	1 = highest level of preparedness	R = Recovery week
▥	Minor peak	2	U = Unloading
▦	Competition	3	
▦	Testing dates	4	
		5 = lowest level of preparedness	

Figure 7.3 Annual training plan for a collegiate endurance runner.

Date	Month	Aug	September				October				Nov
	Week	30	6	13	20	27	4	11	18	25	1

Competition

	Domestic	▓		▓			▓		▓		■
	International										
	Name of competition	Preston Relays		WVU Invitational			Paul Short Invitational		Penn State Open		Big East Championship

Periodization

Training phase	Competitive 1									
Training subphase	Precompetition				Competition					
Macrocycle	Macrocycle 1 (continued)									
Mesocycle	4				5					6
Microcycle	13	14	15	16	17	18	19	20	21	22
Resistance training	2	2	2	2	2	1	1	1	0	0
Endurance training	6	6	6	6	6	6	6	6	5	5
Speed training										
Peaking index	3	3	3	3	3	2	2	2	1	1
Testing dates	▦									
Recovery weeks				U					U	U

Resistance training

Sets x repetitions	3 x 5	3 x 5	3 x 5	3 x 5	5 x 3	3 x 3	3 x 3	3 x 3	0	0
Intensity	M	MH	H	M	MH	H	VH	M		
Strength-endurance										
Basic strength	▓	▓	▓	▓						
Strength-power					▒	▒	▒	▒		
Peaking									▓	▓

Endurance training

Time										
Distance										
Intensity										

Work load

Workload	
▒	Resistance training
■	Endurance training

Intensity zones	
Intensity	**Percent**
Very heavy (VH)	95–100%
Heavy (V)	90–95%
Moderately heavy (MH)	85–90%
Moderate (M)	80–85%
Moderately light (ML)	75–80%
Light (L)	70–75%
Very light (VL)	≤70%

(continued)

Figure 7.3 *(continued)* Annual training plan for a collegiate endurance runner.

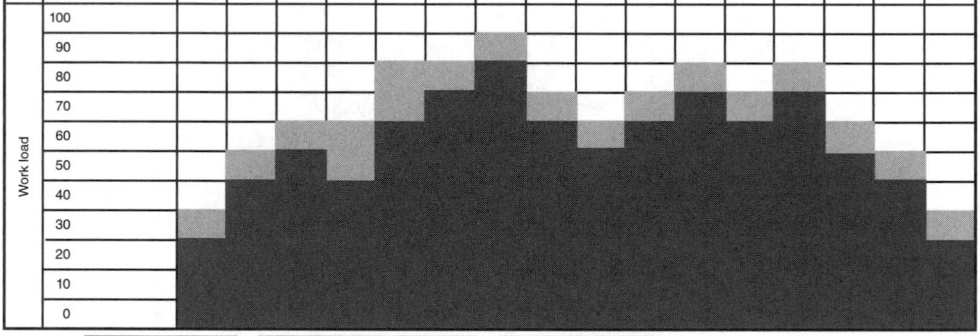

	Month	Feb	March				April				May				
Date	Week	28	7	14	21	28	4	11	18	25	2	9	16	23	30
Competition	Domestic				▒▒▒	▒▒▒	▒▒▒	▒▒▒	▒▒▒		███				
	International														
	Name of competition				Wake Forest Open	WJU Invitational	Princeton Invitational	RMU Invitational	WVU Invitational		Big East Championship				
Periodization	Training phase	Preparatory 3				Competitive						Transition			
	Training subphase	General		Specific		Precomp		Competitive				Transition			
	Macrocycle	Macrocycle 3													
	Mesocycle	12		13			14				15		16			
	Microcycle	39	40	41	42	43	44	45	46	47	48	49	50	51	52
	Resistance training	2	2	2	2	2	2	1	1	0	0	0	1	1	2
	Endurance training	6	6	6	6	6	6	6	6	6	5	3	4	4	5
	Speed training														
	Peaking index	4	4	3	3	3	3	2	2	1	1	5	5	5	5
	Testing dates	▒▒▒									▒▒▒				
	Recovery weeks	R			U					U	U	R	R	R	R
Resistance training	Sets x repetitions	5 x 5	5 x 5	3 x 5	3 x 5	5 x 3	3 x 3	3 x 3	3 x 3	0	0	0	3 x 8	3 x 8	3 x 8
	Intensity	ML	M	MH	ML	MH	H	M	ML				VL	VL	VL
	Strength-endurance												▓▓▓	▓▓▓	▓▓▓
	Basic strength	███	███	███	███										
	Strength-power					▒▒▒	▒▒▒	▒▒▒	▒▒▒						
	Peaking										███				
Endurance training	Time														
	Distance														
	Intensity														

Work load (graph, values 0–100):

Workload	
░░	Resistance training
██	Endurance training

Intensity zones	
Intensity	Percent
Very heavy (VH)	95–100%
Heavy (V)	90–95%
Moderately heavy (MH)	85–90%
Moderate (M)	80–85%
Moderately light (ML)	75–80%
Light (L)	70–75%
Very light (VL)	≤70%

Outline the Basic Structure of the Mesocycles

Once the competitive calendar, the macrocycles, and the phases and subphases have been outlined, the next step is to design the structure of the mesocycles. This step is a little more difficult than creating the macrocycle structure because the resistance and endurance training must be considered in relation to the phases and subphases that have been established. Continuing with the example of the collegiate distance runner, the first macrocycle (which included a total of 22 weeks) can be broken into six mesocycles. Each mesocycle would have very specific targets (figure 7.3).

In mesocycle 1, which is part of the preparatory phase, resistance training is used to target the development of strength endurance; the endurance portion of the training program involves base work. Because the preparatory phase is long, three mesocycles can be established that progress the resistance training from strength endurance in mesocycle 1, to a focus on increasing muscular strength in mesocycle 2, and then a return to the development of strength endurance in mesocycle 3.

The competitive phase is also long (a total of 10 weeks), so it can be broken into three mesocycles also (see mesocycles 4 to 6 in figure 7.3). This phase begins with the fourth mesocycle, which includes 4 weeks of resistance training that targets strength development. Next, the fifth mesocycle contains 4 weeks of training that targets strength and power development. The sixth mesocycle, or last 2 weeks of this phase, is an unloading period in which no resistance training is undertaken in order to maximize recovery, reduce fatigue in the legs, and stimulate a peaking of performance. The development of the mesocycle structures for the second and third macrocycles would progress in a similar fashion. Remember that the various resistance training activities should be sequenced so that the physiological and performance gains are directed toward the specified competitions established in the macrocycle plan.

Construct the Individual Microcycle Plans

After outlining the structure of the mesocycles, the coach can establish the individual microcycles (as shown in figure 7.3). The first step in creating the microcycle structure is to define the number of training days or sessions that will be used for resistance, endurance, and other training modalities. The number of sessions contained in each microcycle will largely be a function of the phase of training and the targeted training goals.

For example, in mesocycle 1, the primary focus of the general preparatory subphase is physical development; therefore, a greater focus can be placed on resistance training. During this mesocycle, the resistance training program will target the development of strength endurance and will be performed 3 days per week. The athlete will perform endurance training activities 6 days a week. A similar breakdown will be used for mesocycles 2 and 3. As the athlete transitions into mesocycles 3 and 4, the number of resistance training sessions decreases, and the emphasis of training shifts toward running performance. As noted previously, the number of endurance training days will stay consistent at 6 days per week during these two mesocycles.

As the athlete begins to shift into the competitive phase (mesocycle 5), the amount of resistance training will be further reduced so that the athlete is performing only one session per week. During this phase, the frequency of endurance training will remain high, but the types of training will vary depending on the targeted goals. Finally, during the peaking phase of the first macrocycle, resistance training is completely removed from the program. This allows the athlete to recover and alleviates the fatigue that has been generated from the training activities.

The second step in constructing the microcycle is to determine the general intensity that will be used for the training weeks and to determine when unloading weeks will occur. The loading program for the individual microcycles can be implemented in many ways. The classic model includes a 3:1 loading program in which the intensity increases for 3 successive weeks and then decreases on the 4th week (see figure 7.4). This basic model is used in mesocycle 1 as shown in figure 7.3; the first 3 weeks include a steady increase in training load, and the 4th week is an unloading week.

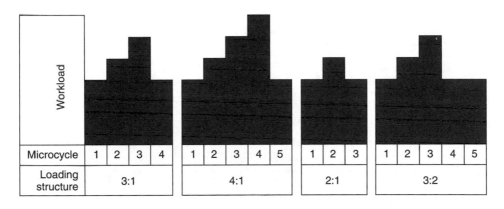

Figure 7.4 Sample loading patterns for a microcycle.

When determining the loading pattern, the coach needs to consider all training factors, including total workload. These factors all contribute to an athlete's fatigue level. Depending on the mesocycle structures, other loading programs can be used, such as a 4:1 or 2:1 pattern (see figure 7.4). Ultimately, the coach and athlete have a lot of freedom to manipulate the loading structures based on the competitive schedule and the athlete's needs.

For the resistance training portion of the program, the average intensity during a microcycle will be indicated on the plan chart. However, this does not mean that the intensity will be constant on each training day. Light and heavy days should both be included, especially when using a combination of training factors, such as endurance and resistance training. Remember that the fatigue from one training factor will affect the athlete's ability to perform the other factor. Research indicates that loading structures that include light and heavy days result in significantly better adaptation because they allow for greater variation in the microcycle. Table 7.11 presents a sample weekly microcycle for a distance runner. In this sample, the average intensity for the microcycle would be classified as very light (VL = less than 70 percent of the estimated 15RM), but each lifting day involves a different intensity (see Monday and Wednesday). By manipulating the intensity of each training day, the coach or athlete can also manipulate the overall volume load, or workload.

Table 7.11 Sample Weekly Microcycle for a Distance Runner

| | Training factor | | |
| | | Resistance training | |
Day	Endurance training	Sets × reps	Intensity (% of 15RM)*
Sunday	Rest day	Rest day	
Monday	45-min fartlek	3 × 15	75-80% (ML)
Tuesday	60-min long slow distance (LSD) run		
Wednesday	45-min interval run	3 × 15	70-75% (L)
Thursday	60-min run over hills		
Friday	45-min repetition run	3 × 15	<70% (VL)
Saturday	120-min LSD run		

*ML is moderately light, L is light, and VL is very light.

Adapted from B.H. Reuter and P.S. Hagerman, 2008, Aerobic endurance exercise training. In *Essentials of strength training and conditioning*, 3rd ed., edited for the National Strength and Conditioning Association by T.R. Baechle and R.W. Earle (Champaign, IL: Human Kinetics), 490-539.

Note that the workload will be multicompartmental and will include contributions from both endurance and resistance training. In figure 7.3 on page 158, this is indicated by two distinct categories being combined to represent the workload. In mesocycle 1, the resistance training will target strength endurance, so the athlete will perform a higher volume of resistance training (3 sets of 15 repetitions). This is indicated by larger bars on the workload graph (figure 7.3). As the athlete progresses through the training year, the volume of resistance training will vary depending on the targeted outcomes. In the plan shown in figure 7.3, a section for endurance training is also included that allows the coach to indicate distance (mileage), training time, and intensity (power output, percentage of maximum heart rate, and so on) for each microcycle. A complete discussion of how this can be distributed is beyond the scope of this chapter. The important message here is that the endurance and resistance training programs need to be treated as a unified and sequenced training load. Refer to chapter 3 for methods of creating endurance training regimens.

Determine the Structure of Training Days

Once the basic structure of the microcycles has been established, the coach can create the daily training structures. When establishing the day's training activities, the coach must consider the various training factors and how they affect each other. As noted previously, the fatigue generated from endurance training will compromise the athlete's ability to perform resistance training if the two sessions are in close proximity to one another. This step involves determining the number of training sessions that occur during the day and sequencing them to meet the goals that have been established for the mesocycle.

Additionally, the coach can determine the intensity of the training sessions. For example, if a hard resistance training session is scheduled for the morning, then the afternoon endurance session would most likely be less intense and may target recovery. Conversely, if a hard endurance workout is planned, then the resistance training session that precedes it would need to be of lower intensity. Once the daily training structures are established, the coach can then design the individual resistance training sessions.

Establish the Individual Workouts

The last step in creating a resistance training program is to design the individual workouts. In this step, the coach must remember the training targets established for the macrocycle, the mesocycle, and most important, the microcycle. These targets will serve as the guidelines for creating each individual workout. Several items need to be included in an individual workout plan, including the goals for the session, warm-up activities, the body of the session, and the cool-down. Figure 7.5 on page 166 shows a sample plan for an individual workout. (This sample training session is based on multijoint exercises that provide a major emphasis on the lower body and only a minor emphasis on the upper body.)

Establishing goals for the workout is essential because the goals will guide the athlete and help him focus on key points. A sample goal for an endurance athlete may be to focus on using proper form for all exercises or to maintain a consistent rest interval between each set. The goals are generally highly individualized and address specific items that the athlete should focus on during the session.

The first part of every workout is the warm-up. The plan should detail the duration of the warm-up and all activities to be performed. Additionally, any distances for activities should be indicated. The warm-up should involve dynamic activities that increase body temperature and range of motion. Athletes should avoid static stretching during the warm-up because this type of stretching has been shown to compromise strength and power performance.

Figure 7.5 Sample Workout Session

Athlete: _Kelsey Fowler_   Date: _2/23/09_

Mesocycle: _1_   Session time: _8:00 a.m._

Microcycle: _1_   Sport: _Cross country_

GOALS

- Focus on the depth of the back squat.
- Maintain technique throughout the session.
- Maintain 1-minute rest intervals between sets.

WARM-UP: 20 MINUTES

- 10 minutes of light jogging
- Lunging for 20 meters
- Skipping for 20 meters
- Shuffling for 20 meters
- Backward running for 20 meters
- Leg swings (long, bent, and side to side)
- Hip rotations
- Shoulder rolls
- Shoulder rotations
- Trunk twists

RESISTANCE TRAINING SESSION

	Target sets			
Exercise	**Sets**	**Repetitions**	**Intensity**	**Comments**
Squat and press	3	15	VL	Use as a warm-up exercise.
Back squat	3	15	ML	
Single-leg lunge	3	15	ML	Make sure knee is at 90 degrees.
Behind-the-neck press	3	15	ML	Maintain control of the bar.
Dip	3	15		Use body weight.
Abdominal exercises	3	25		Use your choice of exercises.
Notes:	Use a 1-minute rest interval between each set. Perform 2 or 3 light warm-up sets until the target loads are hit. All target sets are performed at the same intensity.			

COOL-DOWN

Perform 15 minutes of static stretching that include the following areas:

- Shoulders and arms
- Back
- Hips
- Hamstrings
- Groin
- Quadriceps
- Calves

For an additional warm-up before each exercise, the athlete should perform two or three light sets before starting the target sets. The number of warm-up sets will depend on the intensity being used and the type of exercise. For example, in the sample workout (figure 7.5), the squat and press can be used as a warm-up so that fewer warm-up sets are needed for the back squat. In the workout, the target sets should all be completed with the same resistance. This method initiates a greater stimulus for adaptation, which will lead to a more substantial improvement in performance. Generally, the more complex exercises that involve a larger muscle mass should be performed first; less complex exercises that involve a smaller muscle mass should be performed later in the training session. For example, the power clean should be performed early in the session, and the biceps curl can be performed at the end of the session.

After completing a resistance training session, an athlete should always perform a structured cool-down. The cool-down should include a series of static stretching. The postworkout period is the ideal time for improving flexibility. Most endurance athletes, especially runners, exhibit poor flexibility. Therefore, flexibility training should be included in the cool-down.

SAMPLE ENDURANCE RESISTANCE TRAINING PROGRAMS

All resistance training programs should be designed to meet the specific needs of the athlete. Resistance training programs can be constructed in numerous ways. The program should be designed to target the major movement patterns and muscle groups that are essential to the athlete's sport. In the following sections, several sample training programs are presented. These programs are categorized based on the phase of training outlined in the macrocycle plan. Athletes and coaches should use the information about resistance training and planning in this chapter and integrate these concepts with those discussed in chapters 8 through 11 to develop a training program for their particular endurance sport.

Basic Program for Building Strength Endurance

A basic resistance training program for developing strength endurance should be designed to include a larger overall volume—at least 3 sets and greater than 8 repetitions per set; more advanced athletes may choose to use as many as 10 sets for some exercises (including the warm-up sets). As the number of sets increases, the overall intensity (percentage of 1RM) is lowered.

For most athletes, three training sessions per microcycle are more than adequate. If the athlete is primarily focused on the development of muscle mass, the overall frequency and volume of training could be increased (the athlete could train more than 3 days per microcycle). However, in most cases, this is not the focus for endurance athletes. Therefore, the sample program presented in table 7.12 on page 168 is designed to include only three resistance training sessions per microcycle.

Table 7.12 Sample Basic Program for Building Strength Endurance

Day	Exercises	Target sets*		Intensity			
		Sets	Repetitions	Week 1	Week 2	Week 3	Week 4
Monday	Squat and press	3	10	ML	M	MH	L
	Back squat	3	10	ML	M	MH	L
	Incline bench press	3	10	ML	M	MH	L
	Leg curl	3	10	ML	M	MH	L
	Triceps push-down	3	10	ML	M	MH	L
	Biceps curl	3	10	ML	M	MH	L
	Abdominal exercise	5	25				
Wednesday	Hang power clean	3	10	L	ML	M	ML
	Clean pull from floor	3	10	L	ML	M	ML
	Clean-grip Romanian deadlift	3	10	L	ML	M	ML
	Lat pulldown	3	10	L	ML	M	ML
	Three-way shoulder	3	10	L	ML	M	ML
	Abdominal exercise	5	25				
Friday	Squat and press	3	10	L	ML	M	ML
	Front squat	3	10	L	ML	M	ML
	Bench press	3	10	L	ML	M	ML
	Glute-ham machine	3	10	L	ML	M	ML
	Dip	3	10				
	Dumbbell biceps curl	3	10	L	ML	M	ML
	Abdominal exercise	3	10				

*2 or 3 warm-up sets should be performed with each exercise. 1-minute rest intervals can be used in this phase.

Each resistance training session in table 7.12 is structured to work the total body in one session. This is accomplished through the use of multijoint, large-mass exercises that target movements similar to those seen in most endurance sports. The larger-mass exercises (i.e., squats, hang power clean, and so on) are performed early in each session. This ensures that a minimum amount of fatigue is generated before the athlete performs these technical exercises.

This sample program will last only four microcycles and will use 3 sets of 10 repetitions. Additionally, the intensity will vary for each training day and microcycle. Across the four microcycles, the intensity will increase for three successive microcycles, and an unloading week will take place during the fourth microcycle. This is the classic 3:1 loading pattern discussed previously. To further increase the focus on the development of strength endurance, the athlete can use 1-minute rest intervals between each set and exercise.

This basic program can be used to develop strength endurance, to lose body fat, and to increase overall physical fitness. The basic structure can be used to train for any endurance sport, but in order to maximize its effectiveness, it should be integrated into the overall training structure as discussed previously.

Resistance Training Program for a Runner

The resistance training program for a runner should be designed based on the overall macrocycle structure and the targeted training goals for each phase of training. To illustrate the types of resistance training programs that would fit into a macrocycle training plan, three sample programs are presented based on figure 7.3 on page 158. Specifically, the resistance training plans for mesocycles 3 to 5 are presented.

In mesocycle 3, the targeted resistance training goal is the development of strength endurance. Strength endurance is best developed by using an exercise volume of 3 to 10 sets of over 8 repetitions per set. Therefore, for this phase, the program uses 3 sets of 10 repetitions in order to target the development of strength endurance (see table 7.13). Additionally, the plan for this mesocycle includes only 2 days of resistance training; thus, resistance training will only be performed on Tuesdays and Thursdays. The weekly average training intensity follows the 3:1 loading pattern indicated in the macrocycle plan (figure 7.3). However, this program involves using a heavy day and a light day so that Tuesday is the heaviest resistance training

Table 7.13 Sample Strength Endurance Phase for a Runner

Day	Exercises	Sets	Repetitions	Week 1	Week 2	Week 3	Week 4
Tuesday	Hang power clean	3	10	ML	M	MH	ML
	Back squat	3	10	ML	M	MH	ML
	Dumbbell incline bench press	3	10	ML	M	MH	ML
	Leg curl	3	10	ML	M	MH	ML
	Dip	3	10	Body weight			
	Abdominal exercise	5	25				
Thursday	Squat and press	3	10	VL	L	ML	VL
	Single-leg lunge	3	10	VL	L	ML	VL
	Bent-over row	3	10	VL	L	ML	VL
	Snatch-grip Romanian deadlift	3	10	VL	L	ML	VL
	Pull-up	3	10	Body weight			
	Abdominal exercise	5	25				

*2 or 3 warm-up sets should be performed with each exercise. 1-minute rest intervals can be used in this phase.

day of each microcycle. This loading structure will allow the runner to have harder endurance workouts at the end of the microcycle (Friday through Sunday).

After 4 weeks, the focus of the resistance training program is altered to target the development of basic strength (as indicated for mesocycle 4 in figure 7.3 on page 159). This sample program is shown in table 7.14. To focus on basic strength, the volume is reduced by decreasing the number of repetitions from 10 to 5. Because strength is best developed with higher intensities, the intensity is increased in this phase. As with the strength endurance phase, a 3:1 loading pattern is used. Thus, the third microcycle of this phase (microcycle 15) contains the most taxing resistance training loads, and it is followed by an unloading microcycle. The exercises selected here are designed to maximize the development of muscular strength while allowing for a transfer of training effects that will result in improved running economy. As noted on the macrocycle planning sheet (figure 7.3), resistance training will be performed only 2

Table 7.14 Sample Basic Strength Phase for a Runner

| Day | Exercises | Target sets* | | Intensity | | | |
		Sets	Repe-titions	Week 1	Week 2	Week 3	Week 4
Tuesday	Power clean and press	3	5+5	M	MH	H	M
	Back squat	3	5	M	MH	H	M
	Step-up	3	5	M	MH	H	M
	Push press	3	5	M	MH	H	M
	Dip (weighted)	3	5	M	MH	H	M
	Abdominal exercise	5	25				
Thursday	Power snatch plus overhead squat	3	5+5	ML	M	MH	ML
	Front squat	3	5	ML	M	MH	ML
	Reverse lunge	3	5	ML	M	MH	ML
	Snatch-grip Romanian deadlift	3	5	ML	M	MH	ML
	Chin-up (weighted)	3	5	ML	M	MH	ML
	Abdominal exercise	5	25				

*2 or 3 warm-up sets should be performed with each exercise. 2-minute rest intervals can be used in this phase.

days per microcycle. This allows the focus of the overall training plan to shift toward endurance training and more specialized training typical of the precompetition phase.

The next phase of resistance training, shown in table 7.15, is designed to target the optimization of both strength and power-generating capacity as planned in mesocycle 5 (refer to figure 7.3). In this mesocycle, the focus of the overall training plan continues to shift toward more specialized endurance training. Therefore, the emphasis placed on resistance training continues to be reduced. This can be

Table 7.15 Sample Strength Power Phase for a Runner

Day	Exercises	Week 1			Week 2			Week 3			Week 4		
		Sets*	Repetitions	Intensity	Sets*	Repetitions	Intensity	Sets*	Repetitions	Intensity	Sets*	Repetitions	Intensity
Tuesday	Power clean	5	3	MH				3	3	VH			
	One-quarter back squat plus box jump	5	3+3	MH				3	3	H			
	Push jerk	5	3	M				3	3	VH			
	Abdominal exercise	5	25					5	25				
Thursday	Power snatch	5	3	M	3	3	H				3	3	M
	Step-up drive-through plus split jump	5	3+3	MH	3	3	H				3	3	M
	Clean-grip Romanian deadlift	5	3	M	3	3	MH				3	3	M
	Abdominal exercise	5	25		5	25							

*2 or 3 warm-up sets should be performed with each exercise. 3-minute rest intervals can be used in this phase.

noted by the decrease in the number of resistance training days from 2 in the first microcycle of this phase (microcycle 17) to 1 in the subsequent three microcycles. The overall volume of resistance training is also decreased; the athlete performs sets of 3 with more intensive loads. The increased loads and the exercises selected will result in a further elevation of both strength and power-generating capacity. Plyometrics are also included in this phase. Box jumps and split jumps have been strategically placed in the program in order to maximize explosive strength development. The scientific literature suggests that the inclusion of explosive exercises, such as plyometrics and power cleans, will help athletes develop the strength characteristics necessary for maximizing running performance.

Resistance training is often excluded from the two microcycles before a major competition. The decision to exclude resistance training at this point largely depends on the overall endurance training plan, the level of fatigue generated, and the individual athlete's tolerance to resistance training. If resistance training is used in this mesocycle (mesocycle 6, figure 7.3 on page 159), the training should involve very minimal loads or volumes and should have a moderate to high intensity until the microcycle immediately before the competition. Generally, endurance athletes respond psychologically better to the removal of resistance training during this phase. Therefore, the sample plan focuses simply on endurance training in the two microcycles leading into the major contest at the end of the macrocycle.

Resistance Training Program for a Cyclist

When developing a resistance training program for a cyclist, coaches need to place the primary emphasis on the development of lower-body and core strength; only a minor emphasis should be placed on the upper body. In programs for these athletes, the upper body needs to be deemphasized so that the athletes can avoid an increase in frontal area that would result in a decrease in aerodynamic efficiency. However, the upper body must still be trained because it is involved in activities such as sprinting and climbing.

The structure of the resistance training plan will be based on the phase of the annual training plan and the goals for the individual mesocycles and microcycles. For example, in the general preparatory phase, the resistance training program will contain more training sessions and a larger overall volume of training. Table 7.16 provides an example of a strength endurance phase for a cyclist. In this sample program, the athlete performs 3 sets of 15 repetitions for the major exercises,

Table 7.16 Sample Strength Endurance Phase for a Cyclist

Day	Exercises	Sets	Repe-titions	Week 1	Week 2	Week 3	Week 4
		Target sets*		Intensity			
Monday	Clean pull (from thigh)	3	15	L	ML	M	L
	Back squat	3	15	L	ML	M	L
	Dumbbell incline bench press	3	15	L	ML	M	L
	Dumbbell reverse lunge	3	15	L	ML	M	L
	Clean-grip Romanian deadlift	3	15	L	ML	M	L
	Dip (weighted)	3	15	L	ML	M	L
	Abdominal exercise	5	25				
Wednesday	Squat and press	3	15	VL	L	ML	L
	One-quarter back squat	3	15	VL	L	ML	L
	Bent-over row	3	15	VL	L	ML	L
	Lat pulldown	3	15	VL	L	ML	L
	Standing good morning	3	15	VL	L	ML	L
	Biceps curl	3	15	VL	L	ML	L
	Abdominal exercise	5	25				
Friday	Clean pull (from knee)	3	15	L	ML	M	L
	Squat	3	15	L	ML	M	L
	Dumbbell bench press	3	15	L	ML	M	L
	Single-leg lunge	3	15	L	ML	M	L
	Clean-grip Romanian deadlift	3	15	L	ML	M	L
	Dip (weighted)	3	15	L	ML	M	L
	Abdominal exercise	5	25				

*2 or 3 warm-up sets should be performed with each exercise. 1-minute rest intervals can be used in this phase.

and a 3:1 loading structure is used for four microcycles. Each training session is structured so that the technical, large-mass exercises are done first (when the athlete is the freshest). Additionally, each session is designed to provide a total-body workout that targets the major movement patterns and muscle groups that are used in cycling. To further focus on strength endurance, the athlete can use a short rest interval (1 minute) between sets and exercises in this phase.

When the athlete is transitioning to an emphasis on basic strength (as shown in the sample program in table 7.17), the major modifications to the training program will consist of a substantial decrease in training volume, an increase in the lifting intensity (percentage of 1RM), and an increase in the rest intervals between sets and exercises (2-minute intervals). The reduction in volume load should decrease the fatigue typically associated with high volume loads of resistance training. This will enable the athlete to focus on developing strength and completing endurance-based training on the bike. In the sample program, the number of training days is reduced to 2 per microcycle, and the number of repetitions is dropped from 15 to 5. During this phase, the main focus is still on the development of lower-body strength, which is targeted with exercises such as squats and power cleans. These types of exercises allow the athlete to target the major muscle groups used in cycling while also maximizing the development of core strength without having to perform a wide assortment of exercises.

Table 7.17   Sample Basic Strength Phase for a Cyclist

		Target sets*		Intensity			
Day	Exercises	Sets	Repe-titions	Week 1	Week 2	Week 3	Week 4
Tuesday	Hang power clean	3	5	M	MH	H	M
	Back squat	3	5	M	MH	H	M
	Step-up	3	5	M	MH	H	M
	Push press	3	5	M	MH	H	M
	Clean-grip Romanian deadlift	3	5	M	MH	H	M
	Abdominal exercise	5	25				
Thursday	Hang power snatch	3	5	ML	M	MH	ML
	Front squat	3	5	ML	M	MH	ML
	Lunge	3	5	ML	M	MH	ML
	Snatch pull (from knee)	3	5	ML	M	MH	ML
	Chin-up	3	5	Body weight			
	Abdominal exercise	5	25				

*2 or 3 warm-up sets should be performed with each exercise. 2-minute rest intervals can be used in this phase.

Table 7.18 presents a sample program designed with an emphasis on strength power. To shift the focus toward power development, the overall training volume is further decreased, the intensity of training is elevated, and the rest interval between sets and exercises is lengthened to 3 minutes. The number of training days in this example is held at 2. The low overall volume load of training and the exercises selected, along with the modifications to the rest interval, should help further develop both strength and power. For example, the use of the power clean, power snatch, and speed squat can elevate lower-body power, which should directly translate to power on the bike.

Table 7.18 Sample Strength Power Phase for a Cyclist

Day	Exercises	Target sets* Sets	Repe-titions	Intensity Week 1	Week 2	Week 3	Week 4
Tuesday	Power clean	3	3	MH	H	VH	M
	Back squat	3	3	MH	H	VH	M
	Step-up drive-through	3	3	MH	H	VH	M
	Push jerk	3	3	MH	H	VH	M
	Dip (weighted)	3	3	MH	H	VH	M
	Abdominal exercise	5	25				
Thursday	Power snatch	3	3	M	MH	H	ML
	Speed squat	3	3	M	MH	H	ML
	Snatch-grip Romanian deadlift	3	3	M	MH	H	ML
	Snatch-grip shoulder shrug	3	3	M	MH	H	ML
	Abdominal exercise	5	25				

*2 or 3 warm-up sets should be performed with each exercise. 3-minute rest intervals can be used in this phase.

Resistance Training Program for a Swimmer

Like other endurance athletes, swimmers can benefit from the inclusion of resistance training in their training plans. Typically, swimmers undertake large volumes of swim training; thus, effectively incorporating strength training into their training plans is somewhat challenging. The amount of swim training must be reduced in order to accommodate the number of resistance training sessions or the amount of training load allotted to resistance training.

In the general preparatory phase, a swimmer will usually perform resistance training on 2 or 3 days per microcycle. As the athlete shifts into the precompetitive and competitive phases, the number of resistance training sessions per microcycle will be reduced to 1 or 2. During the 8 to 14 days before a major competition, resistance training may be completely removed from the program. The reduction in resistance training during these phases will reduce the accumulated fatigue and accommodate the potential increase in swim training.

Table 7.19 presents a sample program for the strength endurance phase of resistance training for a swimmer. This sample uses three training sessions per microcycle. The design includes a basic four-microcycle structure that uses a 3:1 loading pattern. Thus, the third microcycle of this phase would be the most difficult. In this example, total-body lifting is used in conjunction with several auxiliary exercises that target the muscles used in most swimming strokes. The overall volume load in this phase is relatively high because of the high-repetition scheme. The short rest interval of 1 minute is used to create additional physiological stress that targets strength endurance.

As the athlete transitions into the basic strength phase, the overall volume load of resistance training is reduced, and the intensity is increased. This is reflected in the sample program provided in table 7.20 on page 176. These modifications enable the athlete to focus on the development of maximal muscular strength. In this phase, the athlete performs more complex lifting exercises, including the power clean and power snatch. Additionally, because the athlete will likely have a greater focus on swim training during this phase, the number of strength training sessions is reduced to two. As with the strength endurance phase, a 3:1 loading pattern is implemented in which the athlete completes three loading microcycles followed by one unloading microcycle.

Table 7.19 Sample Strength Endurance Phase for a Swimmer

		Target sets*		Intensity			
Day	Exercises	Sets	Repe-titions	Week 1	Week 2	Week 3	Week 4
Monday	Back squat	3	12	ML	M	MH	L
	Snatch-grip behind-the-neck press	3	12	ML	M	MH	L
	Straight-arm pull-over	3	12	ML	M	MH	L
	Three-way shoulder	3	12	ML	M	MH	L
	Abdominal exercise	5	25				
Wednesday	Clean pull	3	12	L	ML	M	VL
	Clean-grip shrug	3	12	L	ML	M	VL
	Clean-grip Romanian deadlift	3	12	L	ML	M	VL
	Bent-over row	3	12	L	ML	M	VL
	Abdominal exercise	5	25				
Friday	Overhead squat	3	12	VL	L	ML	VL
	Bench press	3	12	VL	L	ML	VL
	Calf raise	3	12	VL	L	ML	VL
	Lat pulldown	3	12	VL	L	ML	VL
	Front raise	3	12	VL	L	ML	VL
	Abdominal exercise	5	25				

*2 or 3 warm-up sets should be performed with each exercise. 1-minute rest intervals can be used in this phase.

Table 7.20 Sample Basic Strength Phase for a Swimmer

Day	Exercises	Target sets*		Intensity			
		Sets	Repe-titions	Week 1	Week 2	Week 3	Week 4
Tuesday	Power clean	3	5	M	MH	H	ML
	Back squat	3	5	M	MH	H	ML
	Push press	3	5	M	MH	H	ML
	Good morning	3	5	M	MH	H	ML
	Three-way shoulder	3	5	M	MH	H	ML
	Abdominal exercise	5	25				
Thursday	Snatch-grip shoulder shrug	3	5	ML	M	MH	L
	Power snatch	3	5	ML	M	MH	L
	Overhead squat	3	5	ML	M	MH	L
	Chin-up (weighted)	3	5	ML	M	MH	L
	Abdominal exercise	5	25				

*2 or 3 warm-up sets should be performed with each exercise. 2-minute rest intervals can be used in this phase.

After completing the basic strength phase, the athlete may undertake a strength power phase of training. A sample program for this phase is shown in table 7.21. This phase is ideal for the addition of plyometric exercises. The overall volume load of training is again reduced, while the intensity of training is increased substantially. Additionally, the overall number of exercises per session is reduced. The rest interval is lengthened to 3 minutes in order to allow for a more complete recovery before initiating the next set or exercise. This enables the athlete to focus on moving quickly when performing each exercise. The sample program includes two sessions per microcycle, but in some instances, the number of training sessions per microcycle may be reduced to one. The major factor in determining this is the amount of time or effort put into the swim training sessions. If the volume and intensity of swim training are increased during this time frame, then the best strategy is to reduce the resistance training to one session per microcycle.

During the peaking portion of the program, resistance training may be reduced to one session per microcycle—or may be removed from the program—for the two microcycles before a major competition. If one session is included per microcycle, the sessions should contain a reduced number of exercises and a decreased training volume (1 to 3 sets of 1 to 3 repetitions). The microcycle before the competition should include a substantial reduction in intensity; this will help induce recovery while allowing the athlete to maintain strength gains. Again, the decision on whether to exclude resistance training during this time frame will depend on the choices made in the swim training plan.

Table 7.21 Sample Strength Power Phase for a Swimmer

| Day | Exercises | Target sets* | | Intensity | | | |
		Sets	Repe-titions	Week 1	Week 2	Week 3	Week 4
Tuesday	Power clean	3	3	MH	H	VH	M
	One-quarter back squat plus box jump	3	3+3	MH	H	VH	M
	Straight-arm pull-over	3	3	MH	H	VH	M
	Three-way shoulder	3	3	MH	H	VH	M
	Abdominal exercise	5	25				
Thursday	Power snatch	3	3	M	MH	H	ML
	Bench press with medicine ball throw	3	3	M	MH	H	ML
	Snatch-grip Romanian deadlift	3	3	M	MH	H	ML
	Front raise	3	3	M	MH	H	ML
	Abdominal exercise	5	25				

*2 or 3 warm-up sets should be performed with each exercise. 3-minute rest intervals can be used in this phase.

Resistance Training Program for a Triathlete

The integration of resistance training into the overall training plan of a triathlete is probably one of the more difficult things to accomplish. The triathlete must effectively periodize the three major activities of swimming, running, and cycling. Generally, the overall volume of training undertaken by these athletes is substantial and difficult to sequence. Because of the large number of training factors being targeted, the resistance training program must be efficient and contain a minimal number of exercises. The goal is to maximize the physiological adaptations targeted by this type of training without creating too much fatigue. To further facilitate these effects, the coach or athlete must consider the integration of the four training factors: swimming, running, cycling, and resistance training.

During the preparatory period for a triathlete, the resistance training program could include 3 days of training per microcycle, but in most instances, 2 days per microcycle would be more than adequate. Because the triathlete is training for many diverse activities, the best strategy is to divide the daily training into multiple training sessions, as shown in table 7.22. In this example, resistance training is performed on Monday morning and Friday evening.

Table 7.22 Sample Microcycle Structure for a General Preparatory Phase of a Triathlete

Day	Time	Workout
Monday	a.m.	Resistance training
Tuesday	a.m.	Running
Wednesday	a.m.	Swimming
	p.m.	Cycling
Thursday	a.m.	Running
Friday	a.m.	Swimming
	p.m.	Resistance training
Saturday	a.m.	Running
Sunday	a.m.	Cycling

Table 7.23 provides a sample program for a triathlete in the strength endurance phase. This is a general preparatory phase of training, so higher volumes and lower overall intensities of resistance training will be incorporated. Short rest intervals (1 minute) are used in order to maximize the development of strength endurance. Because the volume of resistance training is substantial, the volume and intensity of the training sessions that target swimming, running, or cycling will be reduced.

As the athlete shifts into the basic strength phase, the program will continue to include two resistance training sessions per microcycle. Table 7.24 provides a sample program for a triathlete in the basic strength phase. During this phase, combination lifts will be included, and the overall number of exercises will be reduced. Additionally, the overall volume load of training is reduced, and the intensity is increased in order to target the development of maximal strength. Because maximal strength is targeted, the rest interval is lengthened to 2 minutes so that the athlete has adequate time to recover between sets and exercises. As the athlete shifts into this phase of the resistance training program, the amount of time spent performing swimming, running, or cycling training will likely be increased. One factor that must be considered during this time is the sequencing of the training sessions. Remember, if the resistance training is particularly difficult, the subsequent endurance session must be a recovery session or a session with a reduced training volume or intensity.

Table 7.23 Sample Strength Endurance Phase for a Triathlete

Day	Exercises	Target sets* Sets	Target sets* Repe-titions	Intensity Week 1	Intensity Week 2	Intensity Week 3	Intensity Week 4
Monday	Back squat	3	15	L	ML	M	VL
	Clean pull (from floor)	3	15	L	ML	M	VL
	Behind-the-neck press	3	15	L	ML	M	VL
	Snatch-grip Romanian deadlift	3	15	L	ML	M	VL
	Front raise	3	15	L	ML	M	VL
	Dip	3	15	Body weight			
	Abdominal exercise	5	25				
Friday	Power clean	3	15	VL	L	ML	VL
	Single-leg lunge	3	15	VL	L	ML	VL
	Dumbbell bench press	3	15	VL	L	ML	VL
	Lat pull-down	3	15	VL	L	ML	VL
	Glute-ham machine	3	15	VL	L	ML	VL
	Pull-up	3	15	Body weight			
	Abdominal exercise	5	25				

*2 or 3 warm-up sets should be performed with each exercise. 1-minute rest intervals can be used in this phase.

Table 7.24 Sample Basic Strength Phase for a Triathlete

| Day | Exercises | Target sets* | | Intensity | | | |
		Sets	Repe-titions	Week 1	Week 2	Week 3	Week 4
Monday	Power snatch plus overhead squat	3	6+6	ML	M	MH	L
	Single-leg lunge	3	6	ML	M	MH	L
	Leg curl	3	6	ML	M	MH	L
	Upright row	3	6	ML	M	MH	L
	Abdominal exercise	5	25				
Friday	Power clean and press	3	6+6	L	ML	M	VL
	Step-up	3	6	L	ML	M	VL
	Dumbbell incline bench press	3	6	L	ML	M	VL
	Clean-grip Romanian deadlift	3	6	L	ML	M	VL
	Lat pulldown	3	6	L	ML	M	VL
	Abdominal exercise	5	25				

*2 or 3 warm-up sets should be performed with each exercise. 2-minute rest intervals can be used in this phase.

After completing the basic strength phase, the athlete shifts to a strength power phase of resistance training. A sample program for this phase is shown in table 7.25 (this sample includes one training session per microcycle). In this phase, athletes may use one or two resistance training sessions per microcycle; however, most athletes will use only one session per week because of the increased training time spent on the endurance activities. In this example, the rest interval is lengthened to 3 minutes to allow for additional recovery during the training session. Additionally, the number of exercises in each session and the volume load of training are

Table 7.25 Sample Strength Power Phase for a Triathlete

| Day | Exercises | Target sets* | | Intensity | | | |
		Sets	Repe-titions	Week 1	Week 2	Week 3	Week 4
Monday	Power snatch	3	3	M		H	
	Speed squat	3	3	M		H	
	Snatch-grip Romanian deadlift	3	3	M		H	
	Abdominal exercise	5	25				
Friday	Power clean and push press	3	3+3		MH		ML
	Step-up drive-through	3	3		MH		ML
	Clean-grip Romanian deadlift	3	3		MH		ML
	Abdominal exercise	5	25				

*2 or 3 warm-up sets should be performed with each exercise. 3-minute rest intervals can be used in this phase.

reduced substantially. Volume load is reduced by decreasing the number of sets and repetitions performed during each training session. To ensure that the athlete continues to develop strength and power, the intensity of training is increased. The exercises selected are multijoint, large-mass exercises that provide a very efficient method for enhancing power-generating capacity.

Finally, the triathlete can use a maintenance program. In this type of program, the athlete performs one training session per microcycle. The session would include a minimal number of exercises performed for a low number of sets and repetitions with relatively high intensities. As with the resistance training programs presented for running and cycling, the triathlete may want to remove resistance training from the training plan 8 to 14 days before a major competition. This will enhance the pre-event taper by reducing fatigue and facilitating recovery of the legs. Endurance athletes often complain of having "heavy legs" when they are undertaking resistance training programs. Removing resistance training during the taper appears to eliminate this sensation and enables the athlete to feel prepared for competition.

Running

Suzie Snyder

For endurance runners, improvement in performance is not all about the miles logged and the intensity of the runs. Although these are important, other components of running must also be considered. One component that is often overlooked is running technique. The best runners appear to move effortlessly— they look as though they are moving forward at an incredible rate of speed without even trying. These athletes have perfected their body positions and techniques, which maximizes both efficiency and economy. Running economy refers to the volume of oxygen that the body must consume in order to cover a given distance. In other words, when two runners appear to have equal race performances, one runner may have covered that distance while consuming less oxygen, or using less energy. Running economy is not improved quickly. However, performing technique drills and specific workouts can facilitate efficiency in the way the body moves, which will eventually lead to greater economy.

TECHNIQUE DEVELOPMENT

Technique development is not just for beginners. Seasoned runners will also benefit from performing technique drills. Remember that practicing running technique is different from changing running technique. When athletes perform technique drills, their running style is not radically changed right away. Athletes are simply reinforcing efficient running mechanics, which may gradually lead to positive changes in technique. When technique is less than optimal, athletes may plateau very quickly in fitness. Even when an athlete makes physiological improvements in fitness, the mechanical flaws limit the athlete's ability to improve performance. Many technique drills are also plyometric in nature. Plyometric work is beneficial for muscle strength, strength endurance, power improvement, and strength of bone and connective tissue, all of which are a major part of injury prevention.

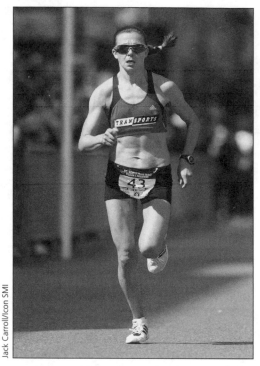

Jack Carroll/Icon SMI

Technique training builds strength and power and prevents injuries in all runners, from beginners to elite-level competitors.

During low-intensity endurance running, the slow-twitch muscle fibers are the primary movers. Therefore, during the base phase of training, which primarily involves low-intensity running, the fast-twitch muscle fibers are used very minimally. As a result of inactivity, the muscle activation potential for these fast-twitch fibers decreases significantly. Restoring maximum potential takes time and frequent power training. To maintain some of the fast-twitch potential without undergoing the stress of high-intensity training, athletes should include technique drills twice a week during the base training phase.

A major part of technique improvement comes from improving neuromuscular communication. This means that going through the motions will not result in improvement. Athletes must focus on performing the drill properly. Here are some factors that athletes should keep in mind when performing all of the technique drills:

▶ **High stride rate.** Stride rate, or the number of steps taken per minute, should always be high, no matter how fast or slow a person runs. When velocity increases, stride length increases naturally, but stride rate only increases slightly. Rather than making each stride longer, athletes should take a greater number of shorter strides to increase stride rate.

▶ **Contact time.** The amount of time that the foot remains in contact with the ground is directly related to the amount of force and power produced from the stride. Time is a major component of power. Therefore, the shorter the contact time, the greater the ground reaction force, stride length, and distance covered with each stride.

▶ **Mid-foot strike.** Heel striking produces a braking effect. Landing on the ball of the foot (also called forefoot or mid-foot striking) allows a decrease in ground contact time; thus, mid-foot striking increases the ground reaction forces, power, and stride rate because of the faster storage and release of energy.

▶ **Vertical bouncing.** Running forward is the ultimate goal; therefore, when a runner's body bounces up and down with each step, energy is wasted.

Athletes should make the most of each stride by moving the center of gravity forward and minimizing vertical bounce.

▶ **Hamstring pull and heel lift.** In the recovery phase, athletes should shorten the pendulum action of the leg by lifting the heel vertically toward the pelvis. A shorter pendulum means a faster pendulum, and a faster pendulum translates into shorter contact time, less vertical bounce, and a higher stride rate.

▶ **Arm action.** The arms counterbalance the legs. The elbows should maintain at least 90 degrees of flexion and should swing forward and back in the sagittal plane, eliminating cross-body swing.

The following drills are designed to help athletes focus on at least one basic skill. Athletes must understand the focus point (intended skill) or purpose of each drill. Many of the drills are plyometric or explosive in nature, so they are best performed on a soft or slightly rebounding surface such as grass, rubber matting, or a hardwood gymnasium-type floor. The drills should initially be incorporated into the base phase of the athlete's training; the athlete can really concentrate on the skills during this phase. Performing the drills a few days each week is sufficient, and some of the drills can be used as a plyometric component of the strength training routine. The overload principle applies here, just as with actual running. Athletes should begin slowly when using these drills. The athletes can gradually increase the volume and intensity as they progress through the base phase and as they become stronger and more efficient.

Step Counting

For 1 minute during a run, the athlete counts the number of times the right foot strikes the ground. The athlete does this several times during the run, aiming for 90 and trying to maintain that stride rate. Athletes who have a low stride rate should try to increase foot speed by focusing on one of the basic skills.

Focus points: High stride rate, Improvement of running economy

Single-Leg Hops

The athlete stands on the left leg with the knee of the right leg bent so that the foot is off the ground. The athlete begins by hopping lightly on the left leg and gradually increasing the heel lift to the point of almost performing a single-leg butt kick. For a more powerful drill, the athlete can perform this action while moving forward, using the free leg to cycle forward and back. The free leg should not touch the ground during this drill. Athletes should begin by performing 5 to 10 hops on each foot; then, after a week or two, they should perform an additional set, gradually progressing to three sets over the course of several weeks. This drill is plyometric in nature, so athletes should focus on landing softly on the ball of the foot with good posture. They should also focus on minimizing ground contact time.

Focus points: Mid-foot strike, short contact time, heel lift, minimal vertical bounce, high stride rate, increased foot and leg strength

Jumping Rope

While jumping rope, the athlete shifts the focus from jumping up and down to simply raising and lowering the lower legs to minimize the distance that the entire body moves vertically. This is difficult to do without scuffing the ground or landing very hard. At first, athletes should try alternating legs, and they can progress to jumping with both legs. The athlete should land softly and stay on the balls of the feet.

Focus points: Foot and leg strength, mid-foot strike, minimizing vertical bounce and contact time

High-Knee Skip

The athlete begins skipping normally and then continues skipping while emphasizing the use of high knees. To emphasize high knees, the athlete leans forward slightly and focuses on lifting the knees with the hip flexors. This drill reinforces the slight forward lean of the running posture and the proper foot strike placement beneath the center of gravity. The drill also helps athletes learn to use fast leg speed and to minimize the vertical motion of the body.

Focus points: Good running posture, increased leg strength, mid-foot strike, minimizing ground contact time and vertical bounce

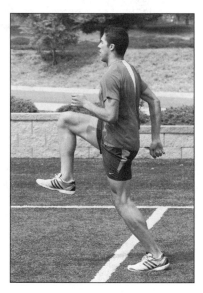

Repetition Skip

The athlete begins skipping normally and then continues skipping while focusing on increasing the number of times the feet touch the ground. The athlete increases this number by only slightly raising the foot off the ground to hop on the opposite foot before replacing it for the next repetition.

Focus points: Lower-leg strength, good posture, minimizing vertical lift of the body while moving the feet quickly

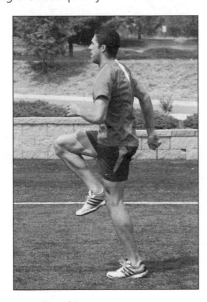

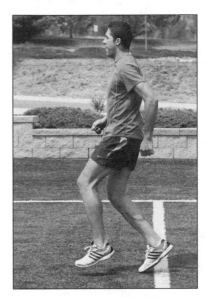

Regular skip.   Skip using low foot raise.

Strides

Focusing on proper technique, the athlete runs for a distance of 50 to 100 meters while gradually increasing speed during the run. The athlete should avoid sprinting in this drill and should not run so fast that the body builds up lactic acid. Between each stride run, the athlete should jog or walk for a few minutes.

Focus points: Training the neuromuscular system to perform with proper technique at faster speeds and integrating all basic components

Barefoot Strides

Athletes perform this drill the same way as the strides drill but without shoes. Locate an area of soft grass and check it for debris before allowing the athletes to run barefoot. In this drill, athletes will naturally land on the forefoot (in order to prevent bruising of the heel) and will limit the time spent on the ground with each contact.

Focus points: Mid-foot or forefoot strike beneath the center of gravity, high stride rate, short contact time

Arm Swings

The athlete sits on the floor with the legs extended straight in front of the body; the arms are bent at 90 degrees at the sides. The athlete begins swinging the arms forward and back slowly. She gradually increases the pace, focusing on pushing the elbows back and keeping the movement in the sagittal plane (forward and back). When the arms swing very quickly, the entire body may bounce up and down. If this happens, the athlete should focus on using core strength to maintain posture and limit any twisting or cross-body swinging.

Focus points: Developing a smooth arm swing forward and back with elbows bent and hands relaxed

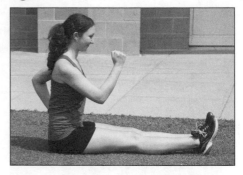

Swing forward.

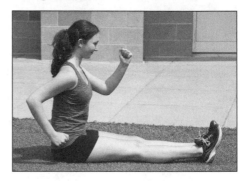

Swing back.

Butt Kicks

This is a traditional track and field drill that emphasizes the rapid hamstring pull. The athlete should allow the hips and knees to flex in order to maintain the range of motion specific to the running stride. While running slowly forward, the athlete alternately lifts the ankle vertically by quickly pulling upward with the hamstring. He begins slowly at first. The athlete can gradually increase foot speed so that he is pulling the heels up very quickly and taking a greater number of steps while moving forward very slowly (fast feet, slow body). The arms must be coordinated with the legs during this drill. The drill can also be done stationary.

Focus points: Mid-foot striking, awareness of using the hamstring to pull the heel upward, maintenance of a high stride rate, practicing the arm swing

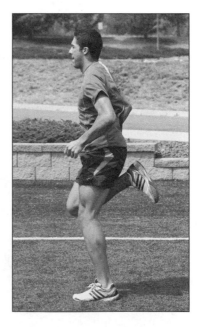

Bounding

The athlete begins by walking, running, or simply taking one or two running steps to build momentum. He pushes explosively off the ground with the back leg, driving the opposite knee up and forward to gain height and distance. The athlete keeps the heel of the driving knee under the hip, ready to land on the ball of the foot. On landing, the athlete immediately drives the other knee up and forward and pushes off the ground with the other leg. The athlete may move the arms in opposition to the legs as in running, or he may use a double-arm swing pattern, pumping with each stride. The arms should swing or drive forward when the leg pushes off the ground and should recover back just before landing to drive with the next takeoff. For this drill, the coach should emphasize the amount of time that the athlete can hang in the air. The more explosive the athlete is, the longer he will be able to hang with each stride.

Focus points: Minimizing contact time, mid-foot striking beneath the center of gravity

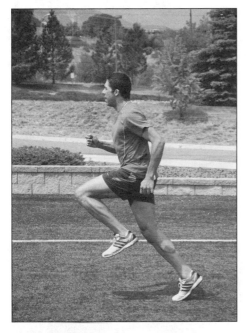

Pushing off.

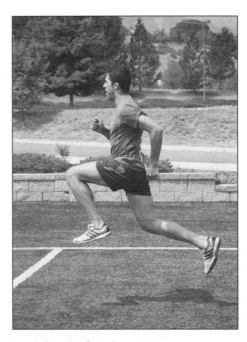

Hanging in the air.

B-Skip

Unlike the actual running stride, the movement in this drill requires that the athlete extend the leg in front of the body immediately after the knee drive phase. Then, the athlete quickly pulls the leg back down to the ground, planting on the ball of the foot beneath the center of gravity.

Focus points: Activating the hamstring in pulling the foot to the ground; planting beneath the center of gravity

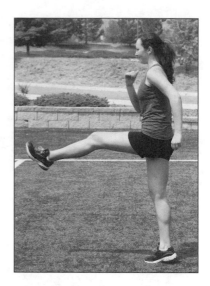

Straight-Leg Skip

The athlete stands on the balls of the feet and begins bouncing from one foot to the other, never lowering the heels to the ground. He continues bouncing in this manner while moving forward by bringing the nonsupporting leg in front of the body, keeping both legs mostly straight. The leg on the ground should have a slightly bent knee, and the athlete should not keep the knees locked out!

Focus points: Planting on the forefoot beneath the center of gravity; coordinating the arms and legs

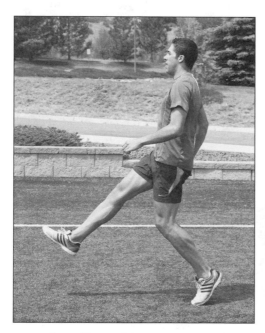

Bouncing off one foot.

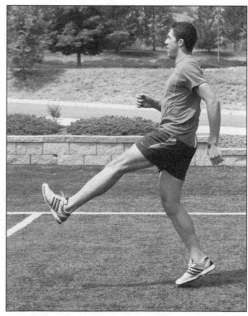

Bouncing off the other foot.

High-Knee Run

The athlete remains on the balls of the feet while alternately pulling the knees up in front of the body. This can be done in a stationary position or while moving forward. The athlete may use a slight forward lean with the torso as well as proper upper- and lower-body coordination.

Focus points: Lower-leg strength, hamstring-activated heel lift, minimal contact time, mid-foot strike, strong arm swings

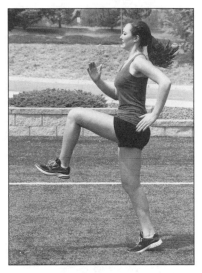

TRAINING PROGRAMS

Coaches and athletes can use the sample training plans in this chapter as a guide when developing training plans for the various distance running events. A sample program is provided for each of the popular events in distance running: 5K, 10K, half marathon, marathon, and ultramarathon. These sample programs can be used to determine the total quantity of running that should be performed each week, including recovery and distance runs. The programs also provide details on the high-intensity workouts to be performed. Technique drills and some distance runs are suggested, but these are not set in stone.

The individuality principle states that each runner will have a different response to the same training; therefore, the sample training plans should be modified to suit each individual's personal needs. For example, total training volume can vary between runners based on personal preferences, abilities, and goals. When designing a program, the coach should always consult with the athlete on these issues in order to create the most effective training program.

Different measures of intensity are used for each sample training program in order to provide examples of the various methods commonly used to gauge intensity. The 5K training program uses rating of perceived exertion (RPE) to measure intensity because many beginning runners start competing at the 5K distance. The RPE measure doesn't require specialized equipment or knowledge, and it is an excellent choice for athletes who do not want an excessively complicated training program. The 10K program uses the Daniels' VDOT system for measuring training intensities. The VDOT system is popular with many running coaches and is included in this chapter to provide the coach and self-coached athlete with some basic knowledge of this popular training system.

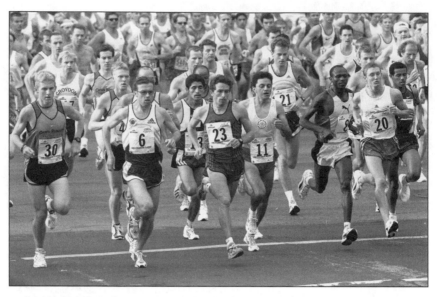

Dedicated training that focuses on individual, personal needs will help an athlete run distance races successfully.

In the half-marathon and marathon training programs, heart rate training zones are used to set running intensities. These zones are also popular in other aerobic or endurance sports, including cycling and triathlon. As mentioned in other chapters, the zones need to be defined so that coaches and athletes both understand the terminology for a particular program. Many coaches design training programs based on heart rate intensity zones, and the athlete must understand how each coach defines each intensity zone.

In the training programs, the higher-intensity training sessions are simply called workouts. These sessions are performed at certain intensities, for a specified time or distance goal, and with specific rest intervals. Remember that athletes need to complete an appropriate warm-up and cool-down before and after these sessions. These workouts are the most important training sessions in the training program because they are designed to produce specific adaptations. Easy distance runs can then be used as recovery sessions. Easy days should consist of runs at a low to moderate intensity that help the body recover; these runs may vary in distance or duration. For the runner who has trouble running every day, the workouts are the important running sessions, and these high-quality workouts should be incorporated into the weekly schedule. These athletes may want to cross-train with nonimpact activities such as swimming, biking, or running in the pool for the easy days. In addition, recovery days are a good time to do technique drills, other active recovery activities (such as yoga), or various passive recovery techniques (such as foam rolling, stretching, massaging, or napping). The athletes should also ensure that they are practicing sound nutrition habits. If athletes are unable to run (or cross-train) on nonworkout days, they should focus on passive recovery techniques. As a general rule, an athlete should take 1 day off for complete recovery every 7 to 14 days.

For athletes who are new to endurance running or who are returning from a layoff or injury, an important consideration is making sure that the training program includes a long enough base phase. The minimum duration should be 4 to 8 weeks. This allows the body to adapt to low and moderate levels of stress in order to prepare for more intense training. If an athlete has a significant running background with a solid base of running fitness, the preparation phase may be significantly shorter. An athlete who has been running recreationally but has not done any high-intensity running should be cautious about the intensity and volume of the initial training. The risk of injury increases significantly if total volume or intensity is increased too quickly. As a general rule, an athlete should not increase total weekly distance by more than 10 percent.

The sample training programs in this chapter vary in duration. When a coach is planning an athlete's training schedule and individualizing one of the sample training programs, the first step is to look at the date of the athlete's event (or most important event). Count back chronologically from the event and plan for the training to start anywhere from 18 to 24 weeks before the event, depending on the length of the base training. One way for a coach to help athletes take ownership of their training is to encourage them to keep a training log. The coach can use this information to track training progress, and it can also help identify a possible risk of injury or illness.

5K Training Plan

The first 6 weeks of training for a 5K should be dedicated to base training (table 8.1 on page 192). In the first 3 weeks, athletes should run at least 4 days per week at an easy pace (RPE 1 to 5) for about 30 minutes each session. The program could include more or less depending on the athlete's running experience. Cardiovascular cross-training—such as swimming, cycling, or pool running—should be incorporated 2 or 3 days per week to supplement the remaining days. In addition, strength training can be done up to 4 days per week along with aerobic training.

For the final 3 weeks of base training, running should increase to 5 or 6 days per week, and technique development drills should be incorporated into three training sessions each week. One session each week should be a long run, which is a low-intensity run of longer distance than any other run in the week (the long run should not be more than 25 percent of the total weekly distance). The athlete continues strength training and decreases cross-training to 1 or 2 days. One day each week should be used for active recovery or cross-training.

Weeks 7 to 12 are considered the first building phase, which means that training intensity should increase; the training will now include 2 or 3 days of hard workouts. The focus should be on increasing foot speed and aerobic capacity using

Table 8.1 5K Training Plan

Training week	Workout 1	Workout 2	Workout 3
Weeks 1-6 **Base**	Base training: Develop an aerobic foundation with 5 or 6 days per week of easy-pace running (RPE 1-5). Perform technique drills 2 or 3 days per week.		
Week 7 **Initial building phase**	• 3 × 400 m at 5K goal race pace with 400 m recovery jogs • 4-6 × 200 m (RPE 9-10) with 200 m recovery jogs	• Hill runs: On a hill that takes 3-5 min to climb, run up 3-6 times, jogging down as recovery the portion. • Goals: strength and aerobic development	• Warm-up • Fartlek: 2 min hard 1 min jogging 1 min hard 30 sec jogging 30 sec hard Jog easy for 2 min • Repeat for a total of up to 5K
Week 8	• 4-6 × 400 m at goal 5K race pace with 400 m recovery jogs • 5-8 × 200 m at RPE 9-10 with 200 m recovery jogs	• Warm-up based on athlete's preferences and needs • Steady 30-min run at RPE 7 • Cool-down based on athlete's preferences and needs	Long run up to 1 hour or up to 7-8 miles at RPE 5-6
Week 9	• 2-4 × 200 m (200 m recovery jogs) • 1-2 × 400 m (400 m recovery jogs) • 1 × 800 m (800 m recovery jogs) • 1-2 × 400 m (400 m recovery jogs) • 2-4 × 200 m (200 m recovery jogs) • All repetitions at RPE of 8-9	• 3-6 × 1 mile at RPE 7-8 with 2-min recovery jogs at RPE 2-4 • Or fartlek 3-6 × 6-8 min at RPE 7-8 with 2-min recovery jogs at RPE 2-4	4-6 × 3-min intervals at 5K goal race pace with 3-min recovery jogs at RPE 3-5

Week 10
Recovery week
Reduce distance
	• Run 2-4 × the following:
	  200 m with 200 m recovery
	  400 m with 400 m recovery
	  800 m with 400 m recovery
	• Intervals at RPE 8-9
		• Warm-up
		• Run 30-40 min at RPE 7-8
		• Cool-down
			Long run at RPE 4-6 about 6-7 miles or 50-60 min

Week 11	• Warm-up • Hill repeats: On a steep hill, run hard up for 1 min or less and then jog or walk down the hill for recovery; run 5-8 reps • Focus: high stride rate, pulling the knees up and forward, and staying on the balls of the feet	• Run 2.5-3 miles at RPE 7 • 3-min jog at RPE 2-4 • 1.5-2 miles at RPE 7 • 3-min jog at RPE 2-4 • 0.5-1.0 mile at RPE 7-8 • Cool-down at RPE 1-5	Intervals or fartlek: • 2 min hard • 1 min easy jogging • 1 min hard • 30 sec easy jogging • 30 sec hard • 2 min easy jogging Repeat for a total of up to 5K (not including warm-up and cool-down)

Training week	Workout 1	Workout 2	Workout 3
Week 12	• Run 3-4 × the following: 200 m with 200 m recovery 400 m with 400 m recovery 800 m with 400 m recovery • Run the intervals at RPE 8-9	Choose from one of the following: • Run for 40-45 min at RPE 7 • Run a 45-min broken threshold run: 20 min (RPE 7) 5 min easy (RPE 2-4) 20 min (RPE 7)	• Long easy run at RPE 5 for about 50-65 min • Count stride rate periodically during the run; aim for 90 strides per min
Week 13 **Final building phase**	Intervals: • 4 min hard (RPE 8-10) • 3-min recovery jogs (RPE 4-5) Repeat for a total distance of 5K	• Warm-up at RPE 3-5 • Run 3 × 2 miles (RPE 7-8) with 2-min recovery jogs (RPE 2-4) • Easy cool-down	Intervals or fartlek: • 2 min hard • 1 min easy jogging • 1 min hard • 30 sec easy jogging • 30 sec hard • 2 min easy jogging Repeat for a maximum total distance of 5K
Week 14 **Recovery week** **Reduce distance**	Run 8-10 × 400 m at RPE 9-10 or race pace with 400 m recovery jogs (RPE 2-4)	• Warm-up • Hill repeats: On a steep hill, run hard uphill for 1 min and jog or walk to recover for 2-3 min; run 6-8 reps • Then run 30 sec on steepest part of the hill with 2-min recovery jogs; run 4-6 reps	• Intervals of 5 min at RPE 7 with 2.5-min recovery jogs at RPE 2-4 • Total distance: 5K
Week 15	• Run 3-5 × 200 m (RPE 9-10) with 200 m recovery • Run 400 m (RPE 9-10) with 400 m recovery • Run 800 m (RPE 9-10) with 400 m recovery	Run 2-4 × 1.5 miles (RPE 7) or race pace with 2-min recovery jog	Long, easy run with race pace pickups: • 30-sec race pace pickups once or twice every 5 min • Jog at least 2 min between race pace bouts
Week 16	Run 6-8 × 400 m (RPE 8 or race pace) with 400 m recovery jogs	• Run for 12 min (RPE 7) • Jog for 3 min (RPE 2-4) • Repeat the 12 min (RPE 7) • Finish by cooling down	• Run 3 × 1 mile (RPE 7-8 or race pace) with a rest time of half your run time for the 1 mile • Finish by cooling down
Week 17	• Warm-up • Run intervals of 4 min hard (RPE 7-8) with 3-min recovery jogs (RPE 2-4); total distance: 5 miles • Cool-down Warm-up and cool-down distance not to be included in the 5 miles	Run 3-4 × 10 min (RPE 7) with 2-min recovery jogs (RPE 2-4)	• Run 800 m (RPE 9-10) with 400 m recovery jog • 2 × 400 m (RPE 9-10) with 400 m recovery jog • 4 × 200 m (RPE 10) with 200 m recovery jog
Week 18 **Race week** **Reduce weekly distance**	• Run intervals of 4 min hard with 3-min recovery jogs • Total distance: 4.0-4.5 miles	Run 4-6 × 400 m at RPE 8-9 or race pace with 400 m recovery jogs	Race

Unless otherwise noted, all recovery jogs are at RPE 1 to 4.
Hard pace correlates to an RPE of 8 or higher.

threshold and interval running. Total distance will increase during this period, but not more than 10 percent every 3 weeks. Recovery is also very important during this period; easy runs and passive recovery techniques should be emphasized. In addition to the high-intensity workouts, easy runs should be included in the schedule. Alternative forms of aerobic exercise may substitute for easy running on recovery days. Swimming, water running, cross-country skiing, and cycling are great alternatives because they relieve the joints of stress while maintaining cardiovascular demands.

For the last 5 weeks of training (weeks 13 to 18), the intensity should be increased slightly by emphasizing running at threshold pace and using intervals of longer duration. For most recreational athletes racing the 5K distance, the taper for competition is built into the training program. The 2 days before race day are used for recovery runs. As part of the recovery runs, technique drills should be used as a means for activating the fast-twitch muscle fibers without causing fatigue.

10K Training Plan

This 10K training plan uses the VDOT system to determine training intensities. (This system was developed by Jack Daniels and Jimmy Gilbert. For more details, see *Daniels' Running Formula, Second Edition* [Daniels 2005].) The VDOT system is a measurement of an individual's running ability based on performance times from a race or field test that are used to create an aerobic score. That score is then used to set specific training intensities in order to produce specific adaptations such as improved endurance, speed, or economy. Training at the right intensity at the right time is an important component of a training plan. Tables 8.2, 8.3 (on page 196), and 8.4 (on page 198) provide VDOT information that is used to develop the sample 10K training program in table 8.5 (on page 202).

The environmental and terrain conditions of each race course will affect VDOT values. Therefore, if the target race will be run on a mostly flat road, the athlete's time from a recent race under similar circumstances should be used in order to get the highest possible VDOT prediction. If the target event will be run on a hilly course or in adverse conditions, then a race run on similar terrain or in similar conditions should be used to get the most accurate prediction. In addition to course and weather conditions, factors such as altitude may affect the athlete's training and racing abilities or performances.

Table 8.2 Types of Training (With Purpose, Intensity, and Duration per Session)

Zone	Purpose	Intensity % $\dot{V}O_2$max % HRmax	Varieties	Duration (min or % of week's distance)
E (easy)	Promote desirable cell changes and develop cardio-vascular system	59-74% 65-79%	Warm-up Cool-down Recovery run Recovery within a workout Long run	10-30 min 10-30 min 30-60 min Up to several min Up to lesser of 150 min or 25% of the week's total distance
M (marathon race pace)	Allow marathoners to experience conditions at race pace; used as an alternative easy pace for others	75-84% 80-90%	Steady run or long repeats	Up to lesser of 90 min or 16 miles
T (threshold)	Improve endurance	83-88% 88-92%	Tempo runs or cruise intervals	Tempo runs: 20-60 min Cruise intervals: repeated runs of up to 15 min each with 1/5 run time for rest; total lesser of 10% of week's distance or 60 min
I (intervals)	Stress aerobic power ($\dot{V}O_2$max)	95-100% 98-100%	$\dot{V}O_2$max intervals	Repeated runs of up to 5 min each with jog recoveries of equal or less time; total lesser of 10K or 8% of the week's total distance
	Stress aerobic system at race pace	Race pace	Intervals at race pace	Repeated runs of up to 1/4 race distance, with equal or less time for rests; total lesser of 10K or 2 to 3 × race distance
R (reps)*	Improve speed and economy	Mile race pace	Pace reps and strides	Repeated runs of up to 2 min each, with full recoveries; total lesser of 5 miles or 5% of week's total distance
		Fast and controlled (race pace or faster)	Speed reps and fast strides	Repeated runs of up to 1 min each, with full recoveries; total up to 2,000 m

*HR cannot be used in R zone because it's not possible to record heart rates greater than 100% of HRmax.

Reprinted, by permission, from J. Daniels, 2005, *Daniels' running formula*, 2nd ed. (Champaign, IL: Human Kinetics), 35.

Table 8.3 VDOT Values Associated With Times Raced Over Popular Distances

VDOT	1,500 m	Mile	3,000 m	2 miles	5,000 m	
30	8:30	9:11	17:56	19:19	30:40	
31	8:15	8:55	17:27	18:48	29:51	
32	8:02	8:41	16:59	18:18	29:05	
33	7:49	8:27	16:33	17:50	28:21	
34	7:37	8:14	16:09	17:24	27:39	
35	7:25	8:01	15:45	16:58	27:00	
36	7:14	7:49	15:23	16:34	26:22	
37	7:04	7:38	15:01	16:11	25:46	
38	6:54	7:27	14:41	15:49	25:12	
39	6:44	7:17	14:21	15:29	24:39	
40	6:35	7:07	14:03	15:08	24:08	
41	6:27	6:58	13:45	14:49	23:38	
42	6:19	6:49	13:28	14:31	23:09	
43	6:11	6:41	13:11	14:13	22:41	
44	6:03	6:32	12:55	13:56	22:15	
45	5:56	6:25	12:40	13:40	21:50	
46	5:49	6:17	12:26	13:25	21:25	
47	5:42	6:10	12:12	13:10	21:02	
48	5:36	6:03	11:58	12:55	20:39	
49	5:30	5:56	11:45	12:41	20:18	
50	5:24	5:50	11:33	12:28	19:57	
51	5:18	5:44	11:21	12:15	19:36	
52	5:13	5:38	11:09	12:02	19:17	
53	5:07	5:32	10:58	11:50	18:58	
54	5:02	5:27	10:47	11:39	18:40	
55	4:57	5:21	10:37	11:28	18:22	
56	4:53	5:16	10:27	11:17	18:05	
57	4:48	5:11	10:17	11:06	17:49	
58	4:44	5:06	10:08	10:56	17:33	
59	4:39	5:02	9:58	10:46	17:17	
60	4:35	4:57	9:50	10:37	17:03	
61	4:31	4:53	9:41	10:27	16:48	
62	4:27	4:49	9:33	10:18	16:34	
63	4:24	4:45	9:25	10:10	16:20	
64	4:20	4:41	9:17	10:01	16:07	
65	4:16	4:37	9:09	9:53	15:54	
66	4:13	4:33	9:02	9:45	15:42	
67	4:10	4:30	8:55	9:37	15:29	
68	4:06	4:26	8:48	9:30	15:18	
69	4:03	4:23	8:41	9:23	15:06	
70	4:00	4:19	8:34	9:16	14:55	
71	3:57	4:16	8:28	9:09	14:44	
72	3:54	4:13	8:22	9:02	14:33	
73	3:52	4:10	8:16	8:55	14:23	
74	3:49	4:07	8:10	8:49	14:13	
75	3:46	4:04	8:04	8:43	14:03	
76	3:44	4:02	7:58	8:37	13:54	
77	3:41+	3:58+	7:53	8:31	13:44	
78	3:38.8	3:56.2	7:48	8:25	13:35	
79	3:36.5	3:53.7	7:43	8:20	13:26	
80	3:34.2	3:51.2	7:37.5	8:14.2	13:17.8	
81	3:31.9	3:48.7	7:32.5	8:08.9	13:09.3	
82	3:29.7	3:46.4	7:27.7	8:03.7	13:01.1	
83	3:27.6	3:44.0	7:23.0	7:58.6	12:53.0	
84	3:25.5	3:41.8	7:18.5	7:53.6	12:45.2	

From J. Daniels, 2005, *Daniels' running formula*, 2nd ed. (Champaign, IL: Human Kinetics), 48-49. Data from J.T. Daniels and J. Gilbert,

10,000 m	15K	Half marathon	Marathon	VDOT
63:46	98:14	2:21:04	4:49:17	30
62:03	95:36	2:17:21	4:41:57	31
60:26	93:07	2:13:49	4:34:59	32
58:54	90:45	2:10:27	4:28:22	33
57:26	88:30	2:07:16	4:22:03	34
56:03	86:22	2:04:13	4:16:03	35
54:44	84:20	2:01:19	4:10:19	36
53:29	82:24	1:58:34	4:04:50	37
52:17	80:33	1:55:55	3:59:35	38
51:09	78:47	1:53:24	3:54:34	39
50:03	77:06	1:50:59	3:49:45	40
49:01	75:29	1:48:40	3:45:09	41
48:01	73:56	1:46:27	3:40:43	42
47:04	72:27	1:44:20	3:36:28	43
46:09	71:02	1:42:17	3:32:23	44
45:16	69:40	1:40:20	3:28:26	45
44:25	68:22	1:38:27	3:24:39	46
43:36	67:06	1:36:38	3:21:00	47
42:50	65:53	1:34:53	3:17:29	48
42:04	64:44	1:33:12	3:14:06	49
41:21	63:36	1:31:35	3:10:49	50
40:39	62:31	1:30:02	3:07:39	51
39:59	61:29	1:28:31	3:04:36	52
39:20	60:28	1:27:04	3:01:39	53
38:42	59:30	1:25:40	2:58:47	54
38:06	58:33	1:24:18	2:56:01	55
37:31	57:39	1:23:00	2:53:20	56
36:57	56:46	1:21:43	2:50:45	57
36:24	55:55	1:20:30	2:48:14	58
35:52	55:06	1:19:18	2:45:47	59
35:22	54:18	1:18:09	2:43:25	60
34:52	53:32	1:17:02	2:41:08	61
34:23	52:47	1:15:57	2:38:54	62
33:55	52:03	1:14:54	2:36:44	63
33:28	51:21	1:13:53	2:34:38	64
33:01	50:40	1:12:53	2:32:35	65
32:35	50:00	1:11:56	2:30:36	66
32:11	49:22	1:11:00	2:28:40	67
31:46	38:44	1:10:05	2:26:47	68
31:23	48:08	1:09:12	2:24:57	69
31:00	47:32	1:08:21	2:23:10	70
30:38	46:58	1:07:31	2:21:26	71
30:16	46:24	1:06:42	2:19:44	72
29:55	45:51	1:05:54	2:18:05	73
29:34	45:19	1:05:08	2:16:29	74
29:14	44:48	1:04:23	2:14:55	75
28:55	44:18	1:03:39	2:13:23	76
28:36	43:49	1:02:56	2:11:54	77
28:17	43:20	1:02:15	2:10:27	78
27:59	42:52	1:01:34	2:09:02	79
27:41.2	42:25	1:00:54	2:07:38	80
27:24	41:58	1:00:15	2:06:17	81
27:07	41:32	59:38	2:04:57	82
26:51	41:06	59:01	2:03:40	83
26:34	40:42	58:25	2:02:24	84

1979, *Oxygen power: Performance tables for distance runners* (Tempe, AZ: Oxygen Power). Reprinted by permission of the author.

Table 8.4 Training Intensities Based on Current VDOT

VDOT	E pace Mile	E pace Km	M pace Mile	M pace Km	M pace 400 m	T pace 1,000 m	T pace Mile	
30	12:40	7:52	11:01	6:51	2:33	6:24	10:18	
31	12:22	7:41	10:45	6:41	2:30	6:14	10:02	
32	12:04	7:30	10:29	6:31	2:26	6:05	9:47	
33	11:48	7:20	10:14	6:21	2:23	5:56	9:33	
34	11:32	7:10	10:00	6:13	2:19	5:48	9:20	
35	11:17	7:01	9:46	6:04	2:16	5:40	9:07	
36	11:02	6:52	9:33	5:56	2:13	5:33	8:55	
37	10:49	6:43	9:20	5:48	2:10	5:25	8:44	
38	10:35	6:35	9:08	5:41	2:07	5:19	8:33	
39	10:23	6:27	8:57	5:33	2:05	5:12	8:22	
40	10:11	6:19	8:46	5:27	2:02	5:06	8:12	
41	9:59	6:12	8:35	5:20	2:00	5:00	8:02	
42	9:48	6:05	8:25	5:14	1:57	4:54	7:52	
43	9:37	5:58	8:15	5:08	1:55	4:49	7:42	
44	9:27	5:52	8:06	5:02	1:53	4:43	7:33	
45	9:17	5:46	7:57	4:56	1:51	4:38	7:25	
46	9:07	5:40	7:48	4:51	1:49	4:33	7:17	
47	8:58	5:34	7:40	4:46	1:47	4:29	7.10	
48	8:49	5:28	7:32	4:41	1:45	4:24	7:02	
49	8:40	5:23	7:24	4:36	1:43	4:20	6:55	
50	8:32	5:18	7:17	4:31	1:42	4:15	6:51	
51	8:24	5:13	7:09	4:27	1:40	4:11	6:44	
52	8:16	5:08	7:02	4:22	98	4:07	6:38	
53	8:09	5:04	6:56	4:18	97	4:04	6:32	
54	8:01	4:59	6:49	4:14	95	4:00	6:26	
55	7:54	4:55	6:43	4:10	94	3:56	6:20	
56	7:48	4:50	6:37	4:06	93	3:53	6:15	
57	7:41	4:46	6:31	4:03	91	3:50	6:09	
56	7:48	4:50	6:37	4:06	93	3:53	6:15	

Times are listed in seconds up to 99, then in min:sec.

E = easy, M = marathon race pace, T = threshold, I = intervals, and R = reps.

From J. Daniels, 2005, *Daniels' running formula*, 2nd ed. (Champaign, IL: Human Kinetics), 52-55. Data from J.T. Daniels and J. Gilbert, 1979, *Oxygen power: Performance tables for distance runners* (Tempe, AZ: Oxygen Power). Reprinted by permission of the author.

	I pace				R pace		
VDOT	400 m	1,000 m	1,200 m	Mile	200 m	400 m	800 m
30	2:22	–	–	–	67	2:16	–
31	2:18	–	–	–	65	2:12	–
32	2:14	–	–	–	63	2:08	–
33	2:11	–	–	–	62	2:05	–
34	2:08	–	–	–	60	2:02	–
35	2:05	–	–	–	59	1:59	–
36	2:02	5:07	–	–	57	1:55	–
37	1:59	5:00	–	–	56	1:53	–
38	1:56	4:54	–	–	54	1:50	–
39	1:54	4:48	–	–	53	1:48	–
40	1:52	4:42	–	–	52	1:46	–
41	1:50	4:36	–	–	51	1:44	–
42	1:48	4:31	–	–	50	1:42	–
43	1:46	4:26	–	–	49	1:40	–
44	1:44	4:21	–	–	48	98	–
45	1:42	4:16	–	–	47	96	–
46	1:40	4:12	5:00	–	46	94	–
47	98	4:07	4:54	–	45	92	–
48	96	4:03	4:49	–	44	90	–
49	95	3:59	4:45	–	44	89	–
50	93	3:55	4:41	–	43	87	–
51	92	3:51	4:36	–	42	86	–
52	91	3:48	4:33	–	42	85	–
53	90	3:44	4:29	–	41	84	–
54	88	3:41	4:25	–	40	82	–
55	87	3:37	4:21	–	40	81	–
56	86	3:34	4:18	–	39	80	–
57	85	3:31	4:15	–	39	79	–
56	86	3:34	4:18	–	39	80	–

(continued)

Table 8.4 Training Intensities Based on Current VDOT   *(continued)*

VDOT	E pace		M pace			T pace		
	Mile	Km	Mile	Km	400 m	1,000 m	Mile	
57	7:41	4:46	6:31	4:03	91	3:50	6:09	
58	7:34	4:42	6:25	3:59	90	3:45	6:04	
59	7:28	4:38	6:19	3:55	89	3:43	5:59	
60	7:22	4:35	6:14	3:52	88	3:40	5:54	
61	7:16	4:31	6:09	3:49	86	3:37	5:50	
62	7:11	4:27	6:04	3:46	85	3:34	5:45	
63	7:05	4:24	5:59	3:43	84	3:32	5:41	
64	7:00	4:21	5:54	3:40	83	3:29	5:36	
65	6:54	4:18	5:49	3:37	82	3:26	5:32	
66	6:49	4:14	5:45	3:34	81	3:24	5:28	
67	6:44	4:11	5:40	3:31	80	3:21	5:24	
68	6:39	4:08	5:36	3:28	79	3:19	5:20	
69	6:35	4:05	5:32	3:26	78	3:16	5:16	
70	6:30	4:02	5:28	3:23	77	3:14	5:13	
71	6:26	4:00	5:24	3:21	76	3:12	5:09	
72	6:21	3:57	5:20	3:19	76	3:10	5:05	
73	6:17	3:54	5:16	3:16	75	3:08	5:02	
74	6:13	3:52	5:12	3:14	74	3:06	4:59	
75	6:09	3:49	5:09	3:12	74	3:04	4:56	
76	6:05	3:47	5:05	3:10	73	3:02	4:52	
77	6:01	3:44	5:01	3:07	72	3:00	4:49	
78	5:57	3:42	4:58	3:05	71	2:58	4:46	
79	5:54	3:40	4:55	3:03	70	2:56	4:43	
80	5:50	3:32	4:52	3:01	70	2:54	4:41	
81	5:46	3:35	4:49	2:59	69	2:53	4:38	
82	5:43	3:33	4:46	2:57	68	2:51	4:35	
83	5:40	3:31	4:43	2:56	68	2:49	4:32	
84	5:36	3:29	4:40	2:54	67	2:48	4:30	
85	5:33	3:27	4:37	2:52	66	2:46	4:27	

Times are listed in seconds up to 99, then in min:sec.

E = easy, M = marathon race pace, T = threshold, I = intervals, and R = reps.

From J. Daniels, 2005, *Daniels' running formula*, 2nd ed. (Champaign, IL: Human Kinetics), 52-55. Data from J.T. Daniels and J. Gilbert, 1979, *Oxygen power: Performance tables for distance runners* (Tempe, AZ: Oxygen Power). Reprinted by permission of the author.

		I pace				R pace	
VDOT	400 m	1,000 m	1,200 m	Mile	200 m	400 m	800 m
57	85	3:31	4:15	–	39	79	–
58	83	3:28	4:10	–	38	77	–
59	82	3:25	4:07	–	37	76	–
60	81	3:23	4:03	–	37	75	2:30
61	80	3:20	4:00	–	36	74	2:28
62	79	3:17	3:57	–	36	73	2:26
63	78	3:15	3:54	–	35	72	2:24
64	77	3:12	3:51	–	35	71	2:22
65	76	3:10	3:48	–	34	70	2:20
66	75	3:08	3:45	5:00	34	69	2:18
67	74	3:05	3:42	4:57	33	68	2:16
68	73	3:03	3:39	4:53	33	67	2:14
69	72	3:01	3:36	4:50	32	66	2:12
70	71	2:59	3:34	4:46	32	65	2:10
71	70	2:57	3:31	4:43	31	64	2:08
72	69	2:55	3:29	4:40	31	63	2:06
73	69	2:53	3:27	4:37	31	62	2:05
74	68	2:51	3:25	4:34	30	62	2:04
75	67	2:49	3:22	4:31	30	61	2:03
76	66	2:48	3:20	4:28	29	60	2:02
77	65	2:46	3:18	4:25	29	59	2:00
78	65	2:44	3:16	4:23	29	59	1:59
79	64	2:42	3:14	4:20	28	58	1:58
80	64	2:41	3:12	4:17	28	58	1:56
81	63	2:39	3:10	4:15	28	57	1:55
82	62	2:38	3:08	4:12	27	56	1:54
83	62	2:36	3:07	4:10	27	56	1:53
84	61	2:35	3:05	4:08	27	55	1:52
85	61	2:33	3:03	4:05	27	55	1:51

Table 8.5 10K Training Plan

Training week	Workout 1	Workout 2	Workout 3
Weeks 1-6 **Base**	Base training: Run at least 5 days per week at an easy aerobic pace. Incorporate technique drills into training sessions at least twice per week.		

Week 7
 	
Increase aerobic capacity, economy, and threshold
	• 4-5 × the following:
	  2 × 200 m at R pace with 200 m recovery jog
	  1 × 400 m at R pace with 400 m jog
		Run 4-6 × 1 mile at T pace with 1- to 2-min recovery jogs between each mile repeat	• Fartlek run:
			  2 min at I pace (1-min E jog)
			  1 min at I pace (30-sec E jog)
			  30 sec at I pace (30-sec E jog)
			• Repeat fartleks for a distance of up to 10K, or a total I pace running time of less than 10% of the week's total distance

Week 8	• Run 10-12 × 400 m at R pace with 400 m E recovery jog (Daniels' suggestion: The total R pace distance should not exceed 5% of the week's total distance.)	Run for 30-40 min at T pace	Long run at E pace
Week 9	• 4 × 200 m (200 m jog) • 2 × 400 m (400 m jog) • 1 × 800 m (800 m jog) • 2 × 400 m (400 m jog) • 4 × 200 m (200 m jog) • All reps to be done at R pace	3 × 2 miles (or equivalent time for your ability) with 2-min E pace recovery jogs	• 5-6 × 3-min at I pace as a fartlek with recovery jogs of 3 min • Make sure that the total I pace running does not exceed 8% of the week's total distance
Week 10 **Recovery week** **Reduce total distance**	4-5 long hill climbs: • On a long hill of 4-6% grade (moderately steep), run at T pace uphill and jog or walk down the hill for the recovery period • 3 min up and recover • 5 min up and recover	Run for 40-45 min at T pace	Long easy run, about 1 hour with 4-6 strides at the end

Week 11	• Run 10-12 × 400 m at your goal race pace with 400 m E recovery jog
	Total repetition distance should not exceed 5% of the week's total distance
	Adjust the recovery runs accordingly
		• Warm-up
		• Run 3 miles at T pace
		• Jog 3 min at E pace
		• Run 2 miles at T pace
		• Jog 2 min at E pace
		• Run 1 mile at T pace
		• Cool-down
			Fartlek run:
			• Warm-up
			• Repeats of the following:
			  2 min at I pace with 1-min jog
			  1 min at I pace with 30-sec jog
			  30 sec at I pace with 30-sec jog
			• Total distance: 10K

Week 12 **Increase lactate threshold**	Short-distance hill repeats: • On a short steep hill (6-8% grade), run 8-10 × 30- to 60-sec repeats with 2- to 3-min E jogs between reps	• 2-4 × 800 m with 400 m jog • 2 × 400 m with 400 m jog in between • 4 × 200 m with 200 m jog between each • 1.5- to 2-min jog between sets • All reps to be run at R pace	Run for 45 min at T pace

Training week	Workout 1	Workout 2	Workout 3
Week 13	For high-distance runners: • Warm-up • 4 miles at T pace with 4 min at E pace • 3 miles at T pace with 3 min at E pace • 2 miles at T pace with 2 min at E pace • 1 mile at T pace with 1 min at E pace • Cool-down For lower-distance runners: • 20 min at T pace with 4 min at E pace • 15 min at T pace with 3 min at E pace • 10 min at T pace with 2 min at E pace • 5 min at T pace with 1 min at E pace • Cool-down	• 6-8 × 1,200 m at I pace with E recovery jogs of 3-4 min • Or, rather than running distance, use the equivalent time: about 4-5 min	• Warm-up • 45-min T pace run • Cool-down
Week 14 **Recovery week** **Reduce total distance**	10-12 × 400 m at R pace with 400 m E recovery jogs	• 2-3 × 2 miles at T pace with E pace recovery jogs of 2-3 min • Or, use time equivalent of 2 miles for your ability	Long hill climb repeats: • 5-6 × the following on a moderately steep hill: 3 min at T pace going up with jogging recovery going down 5 min at T pace going up with jogging recovery going down
Week 15	3-5 sets of 1-mile repeats at T pace with 2-min E recovery jogs	• 4 × 200 m at R pace with 200 m recovery jogs • 3 × 1,000 m at I pace with 2-min recovery jogs • 2 × 400 m at R pace with 400 m recovery jogs	3-4 × 2 miles at T pace with 2-min recovery jogs
Week 16	• 3-4 sets of 1-mile repeats at T pace with recovery jog equal to half of your time for the 1-mile run • 3-4 × 800 m at T pace with recovery jog equal to run time	• Run for 5 min at T pace with 3-min jog • 10 min at T pace with 4-min jog • 15 min at T pace with 6-min jog • 10 min at T pace with 4-min jog • 5 min at T pace • Cool-down	• 2 × 200 m at R pace with 200 m recovery jogs • 2 × 400 m at R pace with 200 m recovery jogs • 2 × 800 m at R pace with 400 m recovery jogs

(continued)

Table 8.5 10K Training Plan *(continued)*

Training week	Workout 1	Workout 2	Workout 3
Week 17	• Run for 10 min at T pace with a 2-min jog • 4 × 800 m at I pace with 400 m jog • 5 min at T pace • Cool-down	Repeat 5-6 × 1 mile at I pace with 3-min recovery jogs between each mile	Long run at E pace with 6 × 30-sec pickups within the run • Gradually increase the pace to race pace • After each pickup, return to E pace for at least 5 min before the next
Week 18 **Recovery week** **Reduce total distance**	• 2 × 2 min hard with 1 min easy • 2 × 20 min at T pace with 5-min jog	• 3 miles at T pace with 3 min at E pace • 2 miles at T pace with 2 min at E pace • 1 mile at T pace with 1 min at E pace	8-12 × 400 m at R pace with 400 m recovery jogs
Week 19	• 2 × 400 m at R pace with 400 m jog • 2 × 2 miles at I pace with 5-min jog • 2 × 200 m at R pace with 200 m jog	Run for 45 min at T pace	Run a 60-min fartlek: • 2 min at I pace with 2-min jog • 1 min at I pace with 1-min jog • 30 sec at I pace with 5-min E jog
Week 20	• Steady run for 20 min at T pace • 4 × 200 m at R pace with 200 m recovery jogs	• Run 3 × 1,200 m at I pace with 3-min jogs • 10 min steady at T pace	Run 5 × 3 min at I pace with 3-min E jogs
Week 21	Run for 40-45 min steady at T pace	Long E run	Run a 60-min fartlek: • 2 min at I pace with 2-min jog • 1 min at I pace with 1-min jog • 30 sec at I pace with 5-min E jog
Week 22 **Recovery week** **Reduce distance**	• Run 3 × 2 miles at T pace with recovery jog or walk of 2-3 min • Or, run 6 × 1 mile at T pace with recovery jog of 1-2 min	• Run 2 × 400 m at R pace with 200 m jog • 3 × 1,000 m at I pace with 400 m jogs • 2 × 400 m at R pace with 400 m jog	• Run 1 mile at T pace with 3-min jog • 1,000 m at I pace with 2-min jog • 400 m at I pace with 2-min jog • 2 × 200 m at I pace with 200 m jog
Week 23	Run for 30 min at steady T pace	• Run 2 × 200 m at I pace with 2-min jog • 2 × 400 m at I pace with 2-min jog • 2 × 800 m at I pace with 2-min jog • 2 × 400 m at I pace with 2-min jog • 2 × 200 m at I pace with 2-min jog	• Run 3 × 1,000 m at T pace with 3-min jogs • 4 × 200 m at R pace with 2-min jogs • 6 × 100 m strides
Week 24 **Race week**	• Run 1 mile at T pace with 3-min jog • 800 m at I pace with 2-min jog • 400 m at I pace with 2-min jog • 200 m (R pace)	Optional workout: • Short, easy run with strides • Or race	Race

Half-Marathon Training Plan

The half marathon is a unique race distance that requires a combination of endurance, strength, and speed. These characteristics can be difficult to balance for the average runner; therefore, running a half marathon demands consistency with training, injury prevention, and recovery. The 24-week training plan shown in table 8.6 on page 207 uses training zones that are based on the physiological lactate threshold, which is the point at which the body cannot clear lactate as quickly as it accumulates. The lactate threshold is critical for endurance athletes because training at or near this point results in increased speed and resistance to fatigue, as well as many additional physiological adaptations. The following training zones are used in the half-marathon training plan:

▶ **Zone 1: Very low intensity, aerobic.** This zone should be used for very easy runs during base training, for recovery runs, and as recovery periods within an interval workout. Zone 1 correlates to a 1 or 2 on the RPE scale.

▶ **Zone 2: Low intensity, aerobic.** Training in zone 2 builds and maintains aerobic endurance and muscular strength and endurance. The term *conversation pace* is often used to describe this level of effort because the runner should be able to carry on a conversation while running at this pace (this is possible because ventilation rate and lactate production are very low). At this comfortable pace, the body learns how to use oxygen efficiently and can become economical. Zone 2 correlates to a 2 or 3 on the RPE scale.

▶ **Zone 3: Moderate intensity, aerobic.** This zone is just slightly more intense than zone 2, making it ideal for base training; however, lactate is produced more quickly as a result of the involvement of fast-twitch muscle fibers. Zone 3 correlates to a 3 or 4 on the RPE scale.

▶ **Zone 4: Moderately high intensity, subthreshold.** The subthreshold zone should stay below the lactate threshold. The threshold zone should correlate to a 5 on the RPE scale. At this effort level, the aerobic system, energy production systems, and slow-twitch muscles are working as hard as possible, placing a heavy stress on the body. The anaerobic energy system has also been triggered to help produce energy, and the lactate that is produced as a result cannot be cleared as quickly as it is produced. Severe fatigue will set in within 1 to 1 1/2 hours if the pace is maintained.

▶ **Zone 5a: High intensity, anaerobic.** The goal of training in this zone is to slightly exceed the lactate threshold in order to develop lactate tolerance and facilitate removal. Interval workouts are important, and the work durations for these workouts can last many minutes (up to 1 hour). Rest periods within an interval session should remain relatively short in order to stimulate continuous lactate tolerance. Recovery periods after these training sessions should be at least 24 hours before performing another session over zone 3. Zone 5a intensity correlates to a 7 on the RPE scale.

▶ **Zone 5b: High intensity, anaerobic.** The goal of training in this zone is to increase anaerobic endurance, develop lactate tolerance, and build fast-twitch muscle fiber. This will involve doing interval workouts in which lactate threshold is exceeded. Work intervals should not exceed 30 seconds in duration, and they must be accompanied by active rest periods of at least three times the work interval. The recovery period after a workout of this intensity should be 2 days. Zone 5b intensity correlates to an 8 or 9 on the RPE scale.

▶ **Zone 5c: High intensity, anaerobic.** The goal of training in this zone is power, speed, fast-twitch fiber development, and muscle growth. To achieve these goals, an athlete needs to perform interval workouts of very short duration at maximum intensities; these workouts should include very long recoveries. Running short-distance intervals at a maximum intensity with a long rest duration stimulates the fast-twitch muscles, anaerobic energy system, and lactate production. Recovery periods after these training sessions should be at least 2 days before performing another workout above zone 3. Zone 5c intensity correlates to a 10 on the RPE scale.

Table 8.6 Half-Marathon Training Plan

Training week	Workout 1	Workout 2	Workout 3
Weeks 1-6 **Base**	Base training: Develop an aerobic base by running at an easy pace 5 or 6 days per week. Incorporate technique drills into three sessions per week.		
Week 7 **Building phase 1**	3 × the following: • 5 min in zone 4 with a 5-min recovery jog in zone 2	Ins and outs: • Begin running counter-clockwise on a track • Run in zone 2 on the curves and zone 4 or 5 on the straights • Run 1 mile in this manner in each direction	• Long run in zones 2-3 • Do not run more than 25% of the weekly distance in this workout
Week 8	3 × 5 min in zone 4 with a 2.5-min recovery jog in zone 2	Track workout: • Run 8-10 × 200 m slightly faster than zone 4 (at about 5K race pace if you know it)	• Long run in zones 2-3 • Do not run more than 25% of the weekly distance in this workout
Week 9	2 × 10 min in zone 4 with a 5-min recovery jog in zone 2	• 6 × 200 m in zone 4 with a 100 m recovery jog in zone 1 • 3 × 400 m in zone 4 with a 200 m recovery jog in zone 1	• Long run in zones 2-3 • Do not run more than 25% of the weekly distance in this workout
Week 10 **Recovery week** **Reduce distance**	3 × 10 min in zone 4 with a 3-min recovery jog in zones 1-2	Track workout: • 4 × 200 m in zone 4 with a 200 m recovery jog in zone 1 • 4-5 × 400 m in zone 4 with a 400 m recovery jog in zone 1-2	• Long run in zones 2-3 • Do not run more than 25% of the weekly distance in this workout
Week 11	Ladder fartlek run: • Run hard (zone 4) for the designated times and easy (zones 1-2) for half of that time • 5 min hard with 2.5 min easy • 4 min hard with 2 min easy • 3 min hard with 1.5 min easy • 2 min hard with 1 min easy • 1 min hard with 30 sec easy • 2 min hard with 1 min easy • 3 min hard with 1.5 min easy • 4 min hard with 2 min easy • 5 min hard with 2.5 min easy	Track workout: • 2 × 200 m (zone 5) with 200 m recovery jog • 2 × 400 m (zone 4) with 400 m recovery jog • 2 × 800 m (zone 4) with 400 m recovery jog • 400 m (zone 5) with 400 m recovery jog • 200 m (zone 5) • Cool-down	• Long run in zones 2-3 • Do not run more than 25% of the weekly distance in this workout

(continued)

Table 8.6 Half-Marathon Training Plan *(continued)*

Training week	Workout 1	Workout 2	Workout 3
Week 12	Fartlek: • 5 × 30 sec in zone 5 then 4.5 min in zone 4 with 1-min recovery jog in zone 1 • The goal is to get the heart rate up quickly in the initial 30 sec, then maintain it for the duration of the interval. • During the recovery jog, allow the heart rate to drop significantly.	Track workout: • 3 × 800 m (zone 4) with 400 m recovery jog (zone 1) • 3 × 400 m (zone 4) with 400 m jog (zone 1) • 4 × 200 m (zone 5) with 200 m jog (zone 1)	• Long run in zones 2-3 • Do not exceed 25% of the weekly distance in this workout
Week 13 **Building phase 2**	Hill repeats: • On a long hill with a relatively low grade (2-4%), run for 4-5 min uphill at the high end of zone 4 into zone 5 • Focus on maintaining posture and a high stride rate • Jog or walk down the hill for recovery	Threshold intervals: • 3 × 10 min in zone 4 • 3-min recovery jog in zone 2	• Long run in zones 2-3 • Do not exceed 25% of the weekly distance in this workout
Week 14	On a track or other accurately measured and relatively flat route, run the following: • 5 × 1,000 m in the high end of zone 4 with 3-min recovery jogs • 5 min of easy running in zone 2 • 3 × 1,000 m in the high end of zone 4 with 2-min recovery jogs	Threshold intervals: • 3 × 10 min in zone 4 • 3-min recovery intervals in zone 2	Variable threshold intervals: • Run for 10-15 min in zone 4, then build up to zone 5 over the course of 1.5 min • Gradually back off and return to zone 4, again taking 1.5 min to do so • Run for another 10-12 min in zone 4 and repeat the interval
Week 15	Hill repeats: • On a long hill with a relatively low grade (2-4%), run for 5-6 min uphill at the high end of zone 4 into zone 5 • Focus on maintaining posture and a high stride rate • Jog or walk down the hill for recovery	Threshold intervals to be done on a relatively flat course where intensity will be consistent: • 4-6 × 6 min in zone 4 • 2-min recovery intervals in zone 2	• Long run in zones 2-3 • Do not exceed 5% of the weekly distance in this workout

Training week	Workout 1	Workout 2	Workout 3
Week 16	On a track or accurately measured course where you can maintain intensity, run the following: • 2 × 1 mile with 2-min jog • 2 × 1,200 m with 2-min jog • 2 × 800 m with 2-min jog • 400 m with 2-min jog Recovery jogs in zone 1-2; intervals in zone 4, rising to the high end of zone 4 by the end of each	Run for 30 min maintaining a high but steady zone 4 intensity	This workout is best performed on a soft surface such as a track, grass, or a dirt trail: • 3 × 2 min in zone 5, then jog for 5 min in zone 1 A relatively flat area is ideal in order to maintain zone 5 intensity.
Week 17	On a track or soft surface such as grass, run the following: • 10 × 200 m in zone 4 with 100 m recovery jog in zone 1 • 4 × 400 m in zone 4 with 200 m recovery jog • 10 × 200 m in zone 4 with 100 m recovery jog	Threshold intervals: • 4-6 × 6 min in zone 4 • 2-min recovery intervals in zone 2	• Long run in zones 2-3 • Do not exceed 25% of the weekly distance in this workout
Week 18	On a track or grass surface, run 6 × 1 mile in zone 4 with 2-min recovery jogs	Threshold intervals: • 3 × 10 min in zone 4 • 3-min recovery jog in zone 2	Power endurance intervals: • 8 × 200 m in zone 5 • 3-min recovery in zone 1
Week 19 **Building phase 3**	• Warm-up: Run 1 mile in zones 2-3 • Run 6 × 1 mile in zone 4 with 5-min recovery jogs • Cool-down: 0.5-1 mile in zones 2-3	Long run: 13-15 miles in zones 2-3	Power endurance intervals: • 8 × 200 m in zone 5 with 3-min recovery in zone 1 • 3 miles in zone 3 • 8 × 200 m in zone 5 with 3-min recovery in zone 1
Week 20	• Warm-up: Run 1 mile in zones 2-3 • Run 8 × 1 mile in zone 4 with 5-min recovery jogs • Cool down: 0.5-1 mile in zones 2-3	• Run 2-3 miles in zones 2-3 • 6 × 5 min at the high end of zone 4 with 4-min recovery jogs in zones 2-3 • 2-3 miles in zones 2-3	• Run 3 miles in zones 2-3 • 8 × 200 m in zone 5 with 2-min recovery jogs • 3 miles in zones 2-3
Week 21	• Warm-up: Run 1 mile in zones 2-3 • Run 8 × 1 mile in zone 4 with 5-min recovery jogs • Cool down: 0.5-1 mile in zones 2-3	Hill repeats for strength: • On a steep hill (6-8% grade), run up for 30 sec, then walk or jog for 1.5 min between each repeat • Run 6 reps	Threshold run: • 60 min in zone 4 as fast as you can (steady) for the duration

(continued)

Table 8.6 Half-Marathon Training Plan *(continued)*

Training week	Workout 1	Workout 2	Workout 3
Week 22	• Run 2 × 10 min in zones 2-3 then 15 min in zone 4 • 2 × 5 min in zones 2-3 then 10 min in zone 4	• Warm-up • Run 4 × 800 m in zone 4 with 3-min recoveries • 4 × 400 m in zone 4 with 2.5-min recoveries • 8 × 200 m in zone 5 with 3-min recoveries • Cool-down: 2-3 miles	Day off
Week 23 **Begin taper** **Reduce weekly distance 5-10%**	• Warm-up: 1 mile in zones 2-3 • 4 miles in zone 4 • 2 miles in zones 2-3 • 2 miles in zone 4 • Cool-down: 1 mile in zones 2-3	• Warm-up: 20-30 min in zones 2-3 • Run 2 × 10-15 min in zone 4 with 5-min recoveries • Cool-down: 10-15 min	Run in zones 1-3 for 5 miles
Week 24 **Race week** **Reduce distance an additional 5%**	Run in zones 2-3 for 45-60 min with 5 × 20-30 sec of strides or pickups within the run	• Warm-up: 2 miles in zones 2-3 • 2-3 × 800-1,200 m in zone 4 with 2-min recoveries • Cool-down: 1-2 miles	Race

Marathon Training Plan

Marathon training demands all components of fitness: high-intensity aerobic and muscular endurance, lactate tolerance, speed, anaerobic endurance, muscular strength, and power. In the program in table 8.7, a large part of the training is focused in the lactate threshold zone in order to build tolerance and push the threshold point higher. By pushing the threshold point higher, the athlete is able to run longer and harder before reaching that point. Hill repeats, long speed intervals, and long runs are very important for developing tolerance to high-distance sessions. Although it may be difficult, logging the training distance will pay off on race day. Typically, speed sessions are scheduled for the beginning of the week when the athlete's legs are less fatigued, and the long run at a slower pace is generally scheduled for the end of the week.

As with all training programs, maintaining a log is helpful for monitoring training. The log helps ensure that training is periodically reduced to allow recovery and adaptation. During the time of recovery (every fourth week in many training programs), multiple recovery techniques may be helpful, including the use of a foam roller.

The training zones used for marathon training are the same as used for the half marathon (page 205). They are based on the physiological lactate threshold.

Table 8.7 Marathon Training Plan

Training week	Workout 1	Workout 2	Workout 3
Weeks 1-6 **Base**	Base training: Develop an aerobic base by running at an easy pace 5 or 6 days per week. Perform technique drills 2 or 3 days per week in addition to running.		
Week 7 **Building phase 1** **Aerobic endurance, lactate tolerance**	Fartlek: • Total duration: 50 min • Warm-up: 10 min in zones 1-3 • Run 5 × 2 min in zone 4 with 3 min of recovery in zone 2 • Cool-down: 15 min in zone 2	• Warm-up • Run 6-7 miles in zones 3-4 on a course with rolling terrain • Allow heart rate to rise and fall with the terrain, but do not drop below zone 3	Hill repeats: • Warm-up • On a moderately steep, long hill (5-6% grade), run up for 3-5 min, staying in zones 4-5a • Perform 5-6 reps of 5-min runs or 8-10 reps of 3-min runs • Jog down the hill, taking 1-1.5 min for recovery
Week 8	• Run 4 × 10 min in zones 4-5a with 3 min of recovery in zone 2 • This can be done anywhere.	On a track or a soft, accurately measured surface, run 5 × 1,000 m in zone 4 with a 400 m recovery in zone 2	Short hill repeats: • Warm-up • On a hill of 6-8% grade (moderately steep to steep), run uphill for up to 1 min • Focus on leg extension and knee drive to produce the most force and power on each stride • Perform 6-8 reps running as hard as you can on each rep, with 2-2.5 min of recovery in zones 1-2
Week 9	Fartlek: • Total duration: 60 min • Warm-up: 10 min in zones 1-3 • Run 8 × 2 min in zone 5a with 3 min of recovery in zone 2 • Cool-down: 10 min in zone 2	Interval pyramid: • Run 2 miles in zone 4 with 400 m recovery in zones 1-2 • Run 1 mile in zone 5a with 400 m recovery in zone 2 • Run 800 m in zone 5a with 400 m recovery in zone 2 • Run 2 × 200 m in zone 5b with 200 m recovery in zones 1-2 • Cool-down	• Warm-up • Run 60 min in zone 4 on a course with rolling terrain • Allow heart rate to rise and fall with the terrain, but do not drop below zone 3
Week 10 **Recovery week** **Reduce total distance**	Track: • 4 × 800 m in zone 4 with 400 m recovery in zones 1-2 • 4 × 400 m in zone 5a with 400 m recovery in zones 1-2	• Warm-up • Run 30 min in zone 5a steady • Finish with a cool-down in zone 2	Short hill reps: • On a hill of 6-8% grade (steep), run uphill for up to 1 min • Focus on leg extension and knee drive to produce the most force and power on each stride • Perform 5-6 reps with 2-2.5 min of recovery in zones 1-2

(continued)

Table 8.7 Marathon Training Plan *(continued)*

Training week	Workout 1	Workout 2	Workout 3
Week 11	Track workout (or other flat, accurately measured course): • Warm-up: 15 min in zones 1-2 • 2 miles in zone 4 with 2 min of recovery in zone 2 • 4 × 1 mile in zone 4 with 1 min of recovery in zone 2 • 2 miles in zone 4 followed by 10-15 min in zone 2 for a cool-down	• Warm-up: 1.5-2 miles in zone 2 • 6 × 5 min in zone 5a with a 3-min recovery • Easy 10 min in zones 2-3 • 10 min steady in zone 5a • Cool-down: 1-1.5 miles • Total duration of workout: at least 75 min	Moderately long easy run: • 1.5 hours or 20-25% of weekly distance • Focus on stride rate, mid-foot strike, and keeping a relaxed upper body • If you feel fatigued, insert a few 20-sec pickups throughout the run (several min apart) to activate the nervous system, recruit more fibers, and break up the monotony of the run
Week 12	• Warm-up: 2 miles easy in zones 1-3 • 4 × 1 mile in zone 5a with 1-min recovery jogs in zone 1 • 2 miles easy in zone 3 • 2 × 15 min in zone 5a with 3-min recoveries in zone 1-2 • Easy cool-down	Track workout: • 6 × 200 m in zone 5b with 200 m recovery in zone 1 • 4 × 400 m in zone 5a with 400 m recovery in zone 1 • 2 × 800 m in zone 5a with 400 m recovery in zone 1 • 4 × 200 m in zone 5b with 200 m recovery in zone 1 • Cool-down	Long run: • 1.5-1.75 hours or up to 25% of weekly distance • Focus on form and count stride rate periodically during the run
Week 13 **Building phase 2** **Increase lactate threshold**	• Warm-up: 2 miles easy in zone 2 • 2 × 20 min in zone 5a with 5-min recoveries in zones 1-2 • 2 miles or 15 min easy to cool down	Track workout: • 4 × 1,200 m in zone 5b with 400 m recovery in zone 1 • 20 × 200 m with 200 m recovery in zone 1	• Warm-up: 1.5-2 miles easy in zones 2-3 • Repeats of 5 min in zones 5a-5b with 2.5-min recoveries in zone 1 for 6 miles • Cool-down: 1-2 miles in zones 1-2

Week 14
 	
Recovery week
 	
Reduce total distance
	• Warm-up: 2 miles easy in zone 2
	• 10 × 400 m with 400 m recovery in zone 1
	• Cool-down: 2 miles easy in zone 2
		• Warm-up: 1-2 miles in zones 1-3
		• 2 × 30 min in zone 5a with 6-min recoveries in zones 1-2
		• 1-mile cool-down
			Long run with fartlek for 90 min:
			• 30 min easy
			• 30 min of the following:
			  2 min hard and 1 min easy
			  1 min hard and 30 sec easy
			  30 sec hard and 30 sec easy
			  30 min easy in zone 1-2
			In this workout, hard means as fast as you can maintain for the prescribed duration.

Training week	Workout 1	Workout 2	Workout 3
Week 15	Track workout: • Warm-up: easy 1 mile • 3 × 1,200 m in zone 5a with 400 m recovery in zones 1-2 • 2 miles in zone 5a with 400 m recovery in zones 1-2 • 3 × 1,200 m in zone 5a with 400 m recovery in zones 1-2 • Cool-down: easy 0.5-1 mile	• Warm-up: 1-2 miles • 2 × 20 min in zone 5a with 3-min recoveries in zones 1-2 • 2 × 10 min in zone 5a with 1-min recoveries in zones 1-2 • Short, easy cool-down	Long run: • Steady, easy pace for up to 2 hours or 25% of weekly distance
Week 16	• Warm-up: 10 min in zones 2-3 • 2 × 35 min in zone 5a with 5-min recovery in zones 1-3 • Cool-down: 10 min in zones 2-3	• Warm-up: 2 miles in zones 2-3 • 10-mile fartlek in intervals of 1 mile: Begin with first mile in zone 5a Second mile in zone 2 Third mile in zone 5a Fourth mile in zone 2 Continue this pattern for the 10 miles • Cool-down: 1-2 miles in zone 2	Day off
Week 17	• Warm-up • On a moderately steep, long hill, run 6-8 reps of the following: 4 min up 2 min of jogging down • Cool-down: at least 1 mile	• Warm-up: 2 miles in zones 2-3 • 40 min in zone 5a • 5 min of recovery in zones 2-3 • 15 min in zone 5a • Cool-down: 1 mile in zones 2-3	• Easy run at steady pace in zones 2-3 • 2-2.5 hours or up to 25% of weekly distance
Week 18 **Recovery week** **Reduce total distance**	• Warm-up: 10 min in zone 2 • 6 × 6 min in zone 5a with 2-min recoveries in zone 2 • Cool-down: 10 min in zone 2	• Warm-up: 1-1.5 miles in zones 1-2 • 4 × 12 min in zone 5a with 2-min recoveries in zone 2 • Cool-down: 1-1.5 miles in zone 2	Long run at steady pace in zone 2 for 18-19 miles
Week 19 **Building phase 3** **Speed endurance**	Track: • 4 × 800 m at race pace with 2-min recoveries in zones 1-2 • 4-min jog in zone 2 • 4 × 800 m at race pace with 2-min recoveries in zones 1-2	Long run: 25% of weekly distance or 18-19 miles	Track: • 10 × 200 m at race pace with 100 m recovery jog in zone 1 • 3 miles in zone 5a • 1-min recovery in zone 1 • 3 miles at race pace

(continued)

Table 8.7 Marathon Training Plan *(continued)*

Training week	Workout 1	Workout 2	Workout 3
Week 20	Track: • 10 × 400 m at race pace with 200 m recoveries in zone 1 • 5-min jog in zone 2 • 2 × 800 m in zones 5a-5b with 2.5-min recoveries in zone 1	Long run: • Lesser of 25% of weekly distance or 15 miles	• Warm-up • 4 miles in zone 5a or at race pace • 2-min recovery in zones 1-2 • 4 miles in zone 5a or race pace • Finish with an easy cool-down
Week 21	Long run: 20-22 miles in zones 1-3	Track: • Warm-up: 1 mile in zones 1-2 • 8 × 200 m at race pace with 100 m recovery jogs • 1 mile at race pace with 400 m recovery jog • 8 × 200 m in zone 5b • Cool-down: 0.5-1 mile in zones 1-2	Day off
Week 22	• Warm-up • Run 3 × 12 min in zone 5a or at race pace with 3-min recovery in zones 1-2	• Warm-up: 2-3 miles in zone 2 • 2-2.5 hours at goal race pace or zone 4 depending on goals • 5-10 min easy in zone 1	Day off
Week 23 **Begin taper**	• Easy warm-up • 2 × 30-40 min at race pace with 5-min recovery in zones 1-2 • Easy cool-down	• Easy warm-up • 2 × 15 min at race pace with 5-min recovery in zones 1-3 • 5 × 1 min of strides • Cool-down	Day off
Week 24 **Final taper and race week**	7 days before race: • 1-1.25 hours easy	6 days before race: • 45 min to 1 hour easy • 4-6 × 100 m or 20-sec strides	5 days before race: • Easy warm-up • 3 × 5 min at race pace with 3-min recovery jogs in zones 1-2 • Easy cool-down
	4 days before race: • 35-45 min easy	3 days before race: • 30-35 min easy • 3-5 × strides	2 days before race: • Day off • Or easy 20-30 min
	1 day before race: • 15-30 min easy • 3-5 × strides		

Ultramarathon Training Plan

The ultramarathon is a unique race in that speed is usually not a goal. For most amateurs, finishing is the primary goal. An ultramarathon can be defined as any race longer than a marathon. The most common distances for ultradistance races start at 50 kilometers (31 miles). However serious ultradistance runners consider 50 miles (80 km) to be the shortest ultradistance race. Some races are 100 miles or more, and there is a category of ultradistance races based on time; 12 and 24 hours are the most common durations for these races. If an athlete is not an experienced runner, then the training for an ultramarathon must include an adequate base training phase. The base phase will likely be longer than those commonly used for shorter-distance events, with a gradual buildup to 50 miles per week or more (see table 8.8).

Many training programs for ultradistance runners include a running-walking strategy during training in order to practice a common race strategy. One training strategy is to set predetermined amounts of time for running and walking, such as running for 20 minutes and then walking for 5 minutes. Another strategy is to walk up the hills and run or jog everything else. These tactics are a great way to plan before the stress and fatigue that will occur during the actual race.

Athletes preparing for ultradistance events must ensure that they have adequate training time. This can be difficult for people with responsibilities such as a job and family life. One suggestion is to perform long runs on back-to-back days. For most people, those days will be on the weekend. The longest training session scheduled in the sample program is 8 to 9 hours over the course of two runs. For most athletes, the time needed to finish the race will exceed the training time, but with adequate training time, finishing is still a realistic goal. As an athlete's goal changes from finishing an event to finishing within a certain time, the training program adapts accordingly, usually with an increased training volume.

Table 8.8 Ultramarathon Training Plan

Training week	Run 1	Run 2	Run 3
Week 1 **32 miles**	Easy run or cross-train: 30 min	Easy run: 4 miles	Easy run: 5 miles
Week 2 **37 miles**	Easy run or cross-train: 30 min	Easy run: 5 miles	Easy run: 6 miles
Week 3 **41 miles**	Easy run or cross-train: 30 min	Easy run: 5 miles	Easy run: 7 miles
Week 4 **31 miles**	Cross-train: 30 min	Easy run: 4 miles	Easy run: 7 miles
Week 5 **44 miles**	Cross-train: 30 min	Easy run: 5 miles	Run at half-marathon race pace: 6 miles
Week 6 **46 miles**	Cross-train: 30-40 min	Easy run: 5 miles	Run at goal race pace: 7 miles
Week 7 **48 miles** **Building phase**	Cross-train: 30-40 min	Easy run: 6 miles	Run 9 miles: • 1-3 easy • 4-6 at goal race pace • 7-9 easy
Week 8 **35 miles** **Recovery week**	Cross-train: 30-40 min	Easy run: 4 miles	Run 8 miles: • 1-3 easy • 4-6 at goal race pace • 7-8 easy
Week 9 **53 miles**	Rest	Easy run: 7 miles	Run 7 miles: • 1-2 easy • 3-5 at 10K pace • 6-7 easy
Week 10 **58 miles**	Rest	Easy run: 7 miles	Run 10 miles: • 1-2 easy • 3-4 at 10K pace • 5-6 easy • 7-8 at 10K pace • 9-10 easy
Week 11 **61 miles**	Rest	Easy run: 8 miles	Run 10 miles: • 1-2 easy • 3-4 at 10K pace • 5-6 easy • 7-8 at 10K pace • 9-10 easy
Week 12 **28 miles** **Recovery week**	Rest	Easy run: 5 miles	• Run 2 miles easy • 4 × 1 mile at 10K pace • Finish with 2 miles easy
Week 13 **58 miles** **Building phase**	Easy run: 4 miles	Easy run: 6 miles	• Run 2 miles easy • 5 × 1 mile at half-marathon race pace 4 min of easy jogging between reps • Finish with 1 mile easy

Jog at easy pace between repetitions to maintain pace.

Run 4	Run 5	Run 6	Run 7
Easy run: 4 miles	Rest or short cross-training (up to 20 min)	Easy run: 6 miles	Long run (easy): 13 miles
Easy run: 4 miles	Rest	Easy run: 7 miles	Long run (easy): 15 miles
Easy run: 4 miles	Rest	Easy run: 8 miles	Long run (easy): 17 miles
Easy run: 4 miles	Rest	Easy run: 6 miles	Long run (easy): 10 miles
• Easy run: 7 miles • 5 × 100 m strides	Rest	Easy run: 7 miles	Long run (easy): 18 miles
• Easy run: 7 miles • 5 × 100 m strides	Rest	Easy run: 9 miles	Long run (easy): 18 miles
• Easy run: 5 miles • 5 × 100 m strides	Rest	Easy run: 8 miles	Long run (easy): 20 miles
• Easy run: 4 miles • 5 × 100 m strides	Rest	Easy run: 6 miles	Long run (easy): 13 miles
• Easy run: 6 miles • 5 × 100 m strides	Rest	Easy run: 10 miles	Long run (easy): 23 miles
Easy run: 5 miles	Rest	Easy run: 12 miles	Long run (easy): 24 miles
Easy run: 4 miles	Rest	Easy run: 13 miles	Long run (easy): 26 miles
Rest	Easy run: 6 miles	Rest	Easy run: 5 miles
Easy run: 7 miles	Rest	Easy run: 15 miles	Long run (easy): 26 miles

(continued)

Table 8.8 Ultramarathon Training Plan *(continued)*

Training week	Run 1	Run 2	Run 3
Week 14 **62 miles**	Rest	Easy run: 6 miles	• Run 2 miles easy • 5 × 1 mile at half-marathon race pace 4 min of easy jogging between reps • Finish with 1 mile easy
Week 15 **65+ miles**	Rest	Easy run: 8 miles	• Run 2 miles easy • 5 × 1 mile at half-marathon race pace 4 min of easy jogging between reps • Finish with 1 mile easy
Week 16 **50 miles** **Recovery week**	Rest	Easy run: 6 miles	• Run 1 mile easy • 3 × 1 mile at half-marathon race pace 4 min of easy jogging between reps • Finish with 1 mile easy
Week 17 **68 miles**	Rest	Easy run: 6 miles	• Run 2 miles easy • 4 × 1 mile at half-marathon race pace • Run 1 mile easy • 3 × 1 mile at half-marathon race pace • Finish with 1 mile easy
Week 18 **72 miles**	Rest	Easy run: 6 miles	• Run 1 mile easy • 4 × 1 mile at half-marathon race pace • Run 1 mile easy • 4 × 1 mile at half-marathon race pace • Finish with 1 mile easy
Week 19 **75+ miles** **Race or peak phase**	Rest	Easy run: 8 miles	• Run 2 miles easy • 4 × 1 mile at half-marathon race pace • Run 1 mile easy • 4 × 1 mile at half-marathon race pace • Finish with 1 mile easy (total of 12 miles)
Week 20 **30-35 miles** **Recovery week**	Rest	Easy run: 6 miles	• Warm-up: 1 mile easy • 3 × 1 mile at half-marathon race pace 4 min of easy jogging between reps • Finish with 1 mile easy
Week 21 **50 miles**	Rest	Easy run: 6 miles	• Warm-up: 1 mile • 6 miles at half-marathon race pace • Cool-down: 1 mile easy
Week 22 **35 miles** **Taper 1**	Rest	Easy run: 2 miles	Run at 10K pace: 3 miles
Week 23 **21 miles** **Taper 2**	Rest	Easy run: 3 miles	Run at 10K pace: 3 miles
Week 24 **Taper 3 or race**	Rest	Easy run: 2-3 miles	Easy run: 2 miles

Jog at easy pace between repetitions to maintain pace.

Run 4	Run 5	Run 6	Run 7
Easy run: 7 miles	Rest	Easy run: 2-2.5 hours or 15 miles	Long run (easy): 3.5-4 hours or 21-23 miles
Easy run: 6 miles	Rest	Easy run: 3 hours or about 18 miles	Long run: 4 hours or 24-26 miles
Easy run: 4 miles	Rest	Easy run: 1.5 hours or about 10 miles	Long run (easy): 3 hours or 20-30 miles
Easy run: 6 miles	Rest	Long run (easy): 20 miles	Long run (easy): 25 miles
Easy run: 8 miles	Rest	Long run (easy): 21 miles or about 3 hours	Long run (easy): 26 miles or about 4 hours
Easy run: 6 miles	Rest	Long run (easy): 26-30 miles or 4-5 hours	Long run (easy): 21-23 miles or 3-4 hours
Rest	Easy run: 3 miles	Easy run: 1-1.5 hours	Long run (easy): 2 hours
Easy run: 6 miles	Rest	Easy run: 15 miles	Long run (easy): 15 miles
Cross-train (easy) for 20 min or rest	Rest	Easy run: 12 miles	Long run (easy): 18 miles
Easy run: 3 miles	Easy run: 3 miles	Rest	Long run (easy): 9 miles
Easy run: 1 mile	Rest	Race or rest	Race or Rest

CHAPTER 9

Cycling

| Neal Henderson

T he sport of cycling includes a variety of disciplines ranging from extremely short and intense track events, to highly variable cross country mountain bike events, to multiday transcontinental ultradistance events. There is no single training schedule that will improve all of the skills needed for competing in each of these disparate events, but some concepts of cycling training are universal. In all cases, being able to generate the highest possible power for the duration of the event is critically important. Other factors that cyclists need to develop include handling skills, pacing, strategy, and team tactics. This chapter focuses on improving endurance cycling performance for both the competitive athlete and the recreational cyclist.

TECHNIQUE DEVELOPMENT

Cycling technique may sound like an oxymoron, but in reality, cycling involves various levels of technique. The circular motion of pedaling the bicycle is one aspect of cycling technique that is somewhat constrained. But how a rider achieves that movement can be altered and trained. Proper bike fit, biomechanics, and rider position have a great impact on pedaling technique. Additional factors such as crank length, pedal–cleat interfaces, and drive train also affect pedaling technique. Regardless of the type of cycling discipline, riders will need to negotiate a wide variety of pedaling speeds (or cadences), forces, and balance requirements during training and competition.

A cyclist must have a fluid pedaling style at both low and high cadences. Specific drills that include efforts both above and below the preferred cadence should be incorporated into the cyclist's training. Research shows that most trained cyclists can perform their highest power output during a sprint at greater than 120 revolutions per minute (rpm). Some sprint specialists are able to pedal in excess of 200 rpm! Athletes attempting to set the hour record in cycling (on a track) typically ride at 95 to 105 rpm, while solo cyclists during the Race Across America (RAAM) typically ride at 60 to 80 rpm. Most modern bikes have enough gear options to allow the cyclist to maintain an ideal cadence regardless of speed.

Comfort at High and Low Cadences

This drill helps cyclists improve their comfort level at high and low cadences. The cyclist starts at the preferred cadence and then adds 10 rpm for 30 seconds to 1 minute while maintaining the same power or speed. Then the cyclist decreases the rpm by 10 from the preferred cadence. The cyclist continues adding and subtracting from the preferred cadence in increments of 10 rpm until there is a break in form, such as bouncing excessively in the saddle. The following provides an example:

- Minute 1: 90 rpm (preferred cadence)
- Minute 2: 100 rpm (adding 10 to the preferred rpm)
- Minute 3: 80 rpm (subtracting 10 from the preferred rpm)
- Minute 4: 110 rpm (adding 20 to the preferred rpm)
- Minute 5: 70 rpm (subtracting 20 from the preferred rpm)
- Minute 6: 120 rpm (adding 30 to the preferred rpm)
- Minute 7: 60 rpm (subtracting 30 from the preferred rpm)

Single-Leg Cycling

This drill is excellent for helping cyclists improve the coordination of the circular movement of the leg through the entire pedal stroke. Single-leg cycling drills are often best performed on a stationary bicycle trainer where there is reduced risk of crashing as a result of the imbalance created. Some advanced riders may be able to perform these drills out on the open road. To start, the cyclist pedals the bike with one leg for 20 to 30 seconds per leg. The cyclist should build up to a minute or more of pedaling with a single leg. Performing several repetitions of this drill at the beginning and end of a workout will help cyclists improve their ability to apply force throughout the pedal stroke. Cyclists do not need to achieve a perfectly uniform application of force throughout the pedal stroke, but reducing dead spots (usually at the top and bottom of the pedal stroke, corresponding to the 6 o'clock and 12 o'clock positions) does improve the pedal stroke.

Cycling Starts

Two types of starts are used in cycling events. In many events, cyclists start from a stop, which requires the riders to be able to select an appropriate gear, get into the pedals, and rapidly pedal up to speed. An excellent time to practice starts is during training rides whenever there is a stop for traffic lights. Athletes should work to be able to click into the pedals without looking at them. This is also a good time to experiment with gearing so that athletes are able to start without excessive weaving side to side while getting up to training pace as quickly as possible.

Handling Drill

Bicycle handling includes being able to ride with the hands on the various positions on the handlebars and comfortably corner, or turn, to both sides with equal confidence and speed. An excellent way to practice this is to set up a line of four to six water bottles in a straight line over 50 to 80 yards or meters in a traffic-free area, such as a vacant parking lot on the weekend. The cyclist practices riding down the line and moving in and out of the bottles as if on a slalom course. The cyclist should start off slowly and gradually add speed. To make this drill more difficult, bring the bottles closer together or offset the bottles to require a bigger turning radius at each bottle.

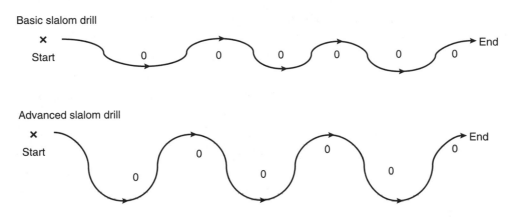

Pack Riding

In most mass-start cycling events, such as criteriums or road races, cyclists need to have the ability to comfortably ride close to other riders. Contact sometimes occurs between riders and their bikes. Being able to react appropriately allows cyclists to stay upright and keep everyone safe in the pack. To improve their pack-riding skills, cyclists should find a large flat grassy area, such as a sport field, and gather several friends to practice riding side by side and in tight formation with one another. The cyclists should practice leaning on each other, touching wheels, slowing to a complete stand, and track standing, or balancing on the bike without moving. These skills make cyclists safer and more proficient in any condition. The safest riders are those who have great balance, never overreact, and are always aware of their surroundings.

ENDURANCE CYCLING TRAINING PROGRAMS

This section provides general examples of training programs for cyclists who are preparing for various types of cycling events. The actual amount of training performed is based on age, training history, competitive level, time availability, and cycling discipline. Some elite professional riders spend in excess of 30 hours per week training and competing during the season. World champions in junior and masters racing categories ride between 6 and 12 hours per week.

However, more is not always better. Training is a balancing act of putting appropriate stress on the body and recovering, which leads to improved fitness and performance. Riders should complete the least amount of training necessary to achieve the greatest response and improvement. Keeping a training log and recording training volume, intensity, perception of effort, and actual performance (including speed, power, and race outcomes) will help determine optimal training levels.

Performing lab or field tests (see chapter 2) is the best way to determine specific ranges of training levels for a cyclist. Coaches and athletes often refer to training zones as a multidimensional evaluation of the training load (see table 9.1). One dimension is actual output, and a portable power meter is the ideal tool for measuring this. Various systems are available, and the most important information that the power meter will provide is the athlete's actual instantaneous power output in watts. Speed is a nice measure of the result of power output, but it is affected by wind, temperature, drafting, and road gradient—making speed a relative marker of output and not an absolute. In comparison, a watt is a watt, regardless of the cycling speed.

The second measure that is typically used for training zones is heart rate. Generally speaking, the more watts produced, the higher the heart rate. The actual heart rate value at a given effort level will vary quite a bit from one person to the next, but defining heart rate ranges from testing will make the use of a heart rate monitor more effective in training.

Table 9.1 Training Zones

Zone	RPE (0-10)	Heart rate (% max)	Power (% threshold)	Duration
Active recovery	0-1	<60%	<50%	20-60 min
Basic endurance	1-3	60-75%	55-80%	1-6+ hours
Aerobic endurance	3-4	80-85%	80-90%	1-3+ hours
Tempo	4-6	85-88%	90-98%	20-60 min
Threshold	6-8	89-93%	99-108%	3-10 min
$\dot{V}O_2$	8-10	94-100%	109-140%	1/2-4 min
Anaerobic capacity (AC)	Variable	Variable	141-200%	10-60 sec
Peak neuromuscular power (PNP)	Variable	Variable	>200%	3-15 sec

A third method of determining training zones is to use a rating of perceived effort (RPE) scale such as Borg's CR10 scale. The CR10 scale ranges from 0 to 10, where 0 is no effort and 10 is a maximal effort. A submaximal effort could be used as the reference point to see how these three methods of determining training zones relate. The level that is very strongly related to endurance cycling performance is a sustainable power that can be held for 30 to 60 minutes in well-trained cyclists. This point is called the threshold, and it typically occurs between a 6 and 8 on the CR10 scale. This point is also typically between 85 and 90 percent of actual maximum heart rate (not estimated maximum).

Another factor to consider when developing a training program is the concept of periodization. Generally, a properly designed program will begin with more emphasis on general fitness and endurance and will then move toward more specific and intense training. The duration of each phase depends on many factors, but the greatest and most sustainable gains in fitness usually occur when an appropriate early-season foundation or base training phase is incorporated and lasts more than 8 weeks. Approximately 60 to 70 percent of the potential improvements typically occur during this base phase of training. The more intensive phase of training usually improves fitness by an additional 20 to 30 percent, and good peaking and tapering yield another 5 to 10 percent improvement.

Many young and professional athletes do very well with a standard 3 weeks of progressive training and then 1 week of a decreased training pattern; however, most masters athletes and athletes with a job, family, and other responsibilities typically achieve greater results with just 2 weeks of progressive training followed by a week of reduced training volume and intensity. The sections that follow provide sample weekly training plans for the preparation (or base) phase of training as well as the intensive build (precompetitive) phase of training. Working with a coach who is certified by USA Cycling is also a good way to devise a personal training schedule that is tailored to strengths, weaknesses, and cycling goals. Joining a local racing club or team is another great way to learn more about the technical and tactical skills necessary in order to perform better and move up through the racing categories.

Road Cycling Training Program

Road cycling typically involves a mix of disciplines including time trials, hill climbs, criteriums, and road races. Some races will include just one of these options, while stage races and omniums will involve some combination of these races. Tables 9.2 and 9.3 on page 227 provide sample weekly plans for the base and intense build phase for riders training to participate in any of these events.

Time trials and hill climbs are the simplest types of races. The distance of a time trial or hill climb may vary, but riders usually use fewer tactics in these race

Table 9.2 Weekly Training During the Base or Foundation Phase

Monday	Rest or active recovery (30 min)
Tuesday	Basic endurance with cornering drills (120 min)
Wednesday	Aerobic endurance (180 min)
Thursday	Basic endurance with 4 × 30 sec of single-leg drills (90 min)
Friday	Cross-training at active recovery intensity (60 min)
Saturday	Basic endurance (5 hours)
Sunday	Cross-training or aerobic endurance ride (120 min)

Table 9.3 Weekly Training During the Intense Build or Precompetitive Phase

Monday	Rest or active recovery (30 min)
Tuesday	Aerobic endurance with 10 × 30-sec cadence builds from 90 to 120 rpm at $\dot{V}O_2$ intensity (90 min)
Wednesday	Basic endurance with 3 × 10 min at tempo to threshold intensity; 3-min recovery (120 min)
Thursday	Active recovery (45 min)
Friday	Aerobic endurance on time-trial bike (90 min)
Saturday	Team ride at aerobic endurance to threshold intensity (4 hours)
Sunday	Basic endurance ride with 10 × 10-sec anaerobic capacity sprints with 50 sec of recovery between sprints (120 min)

formats than in the others. In these races, the goal is to go as fast as possible from point A to point B. Most time trials are between 10 and 25 miles (16 and 40 km) in length, though races can be shorter or longer. In a time trial, riders start at specific intervals, typically 20 to 60 seconds apart. Drafting is not allowed during a time trial, and riders often use specialized aerodynamic equipment, clothing, and helmets.

Time-trial riders are typically larger and stronger bike racers who can push a high power output while keeping themselves mentally engaged and motivated for the entire event.

In a hill climb, riders may use some tactics or strategy based on the profile of the race or the presence of teammates, but this event is still primarily a test of muscle endurance. Hill climbs are the ideal race for riders with a slighter build because this race requires the ability to have a high power output along with low body and bike weight. To determine their uphill racing potential, many riders consider their ratio of power output to body weight. Calculating the rate of vertical ascent (in meters or feet per hour) is another way to categorize a rider's hill-climbing fitness and performance. Top-level professional riders often sustain power outputs in excess of 6 watts per kilogram of body weight during a 20-minute climbing section of a race. Top professional cyclists can also ascend at a rate of 1,800 vertical meters per hour during a fast ascent on a steep gradient. That is greater than a vertical mile every hour!

For cyclists who want to improve their performance in time trials or hill climbs, training typically focuses on increasing basic endurance, improving the ability to sustain a hard effort for long periods, and improving lactate threshold and $\dot{V}O_2$max (by performing intervals). Time trialists and hill-climbing specialists have little need for sprint-type training, but if the goal is overall cycling performance, then this type of training should also be incorporated into the program.

Athletes who compete in criteriums and road races need to be more comfortable riding in packs. They also need to be able to push more intense efforts and recover rapidly between efforts. These riders should perform basic endurance and threshold training (similar to the time trialists and hill climbers), but they also need more emphasis on $\dot{V}O_2$, anaerobic capacity, and peak neuromuscular training.

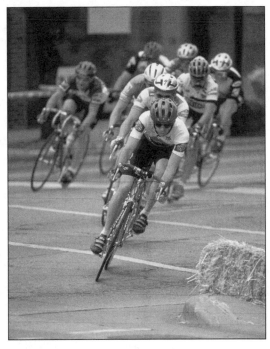

Road cyclists use a combination of high intensity and endurance training in order to adapt to different types of races and situations.

Track and Velodrome Cycling Programs

Cycling competitions that take place on cycling-specific banked tracks, called velodromes, are typically divided into sprint competitions and endurance competitions. Many amateur athletes who have access to a track will maximize their competitive opportunities by competing in various events ranging from sprint to endurance events. The athletes who are most concerned about performance will likely be more specific in their event choices in order to maximize training effect. Track cycling became popular in the late 1800s, and it continues to be an exciting part of the Olympic cycling program. The endurance competitions in track cycling include the individual pursuit, team pursuit, scratch race, points race, and Madison.

For endurance riders, the classic race is the individual pursuit. In international and Olympic competition, men race 4,000 meters, and women race 3,000 meters. The pursuit involves a qualifying round and then a final round. The riders with the top four times from the qualifying round are entered in the finals; the riders with the two fastest qualifying times will compete for gold and silver, while the third and fourth fastest riders in the qualifying round will compete for bronze. The pursuit gets its name from the fact that two riders are on the track at the same time—they start at opposite sides of the track at the same time. In a race final, if a rider overtakes or catches the opposing rider, then that rider wins and the competition is over. At the Olympics, the pursuit includes a qualifying, semifinal, and final round of competition; at all other competitions, this event includes just a qualifying and final round. The team pursuit event is very similar to the individual pursuit, but a team of four riders covers the race distance. For the team pursuit, the current world-record time for 4,000 meters is 3:53.314, which is an average speed of 38 miles (61.1 km) per hour!

The scratch race is a mass-start race with more than 30 riders competing to be the first rider across the finish line after a predetermined number of laps. The points race is typically a 40- to 50-kilometer race that awards points every 5 or 10 laps to the first 4 riders across the line at each intermediate sprint. Any riders who lap the field also receive a large point bonus. The winner of the points race will often not even contest the final sprint if he has enough points. The Madison is a paired points race in which a team of two riders alternate their position in the race by exchanging places with a hand sling every few laps throughout the race. This is a technically and tactically demanding race format that requires incredible focus and teamwork to achieve success.

Most endurance track riders also compete in road racing events. Tables 9.4 and 9.5 provide sample training programs for sprint and endurance track cyclists during the base and precompetitive training cycles.

Table 9.4 Weekly Training During the Base or Foundation Phase

Day of the week	Sprinter	Endurance rider
Monday	Rest or active recovery (30 min)	Rest or active recovery (30 min)
Tuesday	Basic endurance and standing starts (90 min)	Basic endurance (120 min)
Wednesday	Anaerobic capacity sprints (90 min)	4 × 10-min threshold intervals (120 min)
Thursday	Basic endurance (180 min)	Basic endurance (300 min)
Friday	Active recovery (60 min)	Active recovery (60 min)
Saturday	Flying 200M practice (90 min)	Motorpacing* at tempo intensity (180 min)
Sunday	Aerobic endurance ride (90 min)	Aerobic endurance with PNP sprints (120 min)

*Motorpacing refers to drafting behind a vehicle, typically a motorcycle or scooter.

Table 9.5 Weekly Training During the Intense Build or Precompetitive Phase

Day of the week	Sprinter	Endurance rider
Monday	Rest or active recovery (30 min)	Rest or active recovery (30 min)
Tuesday	Aerobic endurance and standing starts (90 min)	Aerobic endurance and AC sprints (120 min)
Wednesday	Keirin competition simulation (90 min)	10 × 2-min $\dot{V}O_2$ intervals (90 min)
Thursday	Aerobic endurance (120 min)	Basic endurance with 30 min at tempo intensity (240 min)
Friday	10 × 1-min $\dot{V}O_2$ intervals (90 min)	Active recovery (60 min)
Saturday	Team sprint practice (120 min)	Points or Madison race (120 min)
Sunday	Basic endurance ride (90 min)	Team pursuit practice at threshold intensity (120 min)

Off-Road Bike Training

Proper preparation for mountain and off-road bike competitions includes training to develop fitness, improve handling skills, and increase speed on downhill sections. Mountain biking is one of the most demanding disciplines in cycling because it requires extremely high levels of fitness as well as highly tuned skills and coordination.

Mountain bike races may be cross country endurance races that last 2 to 3 hours, or they may be short and fast short-track races (like a criterium on trails) that take

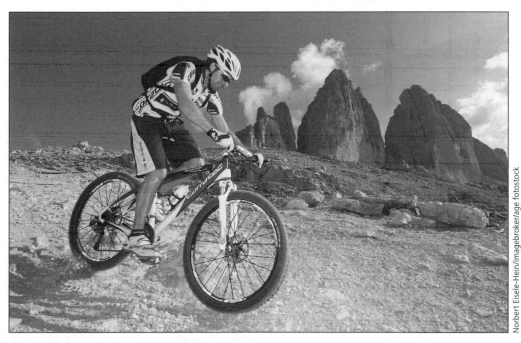

Norbert Eisele-Hein/imagebroker/age fotostock

Mountain bikers must train endurance, handling skills, and downhill speed.

20 to 30 minutes to complete. Mountain biking also includes gravity events such as downhill and four-cross competitions, which typically take 1 to 4 minutes to complete. BMX has also entered the Olympic cycling program as of the Beijing Games. BMX is a short and fast circuit that includes massive bermed turns and large jumps over a course that takes 30 to 40 seconds to complete. Cyclocross racing is also a hybrid style of off-road racing on bicycles that look like a mix between a road bike and mountain bike. These races typically last about an hour.

Most mountain bike riders spend a large portion of their training time on road bikes or on roads because it is easier to control the effort for a ride on roads as opposed to trails. Most elite-level mountain bike riders only spend 20 to 30 percent of their training time riding trails; the remainder is spent on the road developing fitness. Training to be a successful off-road racer will require specific workouts that are designed to improve bike-handling skills, descending ability, balance, and confidence. Most mountain bike events are mass-start events, so being able to start fast and then settle into a rhythm is an important training consideration.

Most cross country courses are made up of a long loop with steep climbs and descents, or racers may ride multiple laps of a course with uphill and downhill segments. On short-track courses, racers typically only take 3 to 4 minutes to complete a lap. These courses include smaller hills than those found on a cross country course—but that doesn't make them any easier.

Most cyclocross courses are a mix of dirt, grass, sand, and even paved surfaces. A cyclocross course is also interspersed with tight turns, obstacles (called barriers) that force riders to dismount and carry their bikes, and short and steep uphill segments. Downhill racers are the daredevils of the mountain biking world. These riders often wear full-body pads and full-face helmets to reduce the chance of serious injury from the inevitable falls that occur in training and racing. BMX is a supercharged sprint that requires incredible acceleration out of the gate, along with confident and skillful bike handling in tight groups. Some of the most powerful riders (measured in sprint power) are BMX riders, and they often score better in peak power output than sprint track cyclists.

Tables 9.6 and 9.7 provide examples of training schedules to be used during the foundation and precompetition weeks for an off-road cyclist preparing for short-track and cross country mountain bike racing.

Table 9.6 Weekly Training During the Base or Foundation Phase

Monday	Rest or active recovery (30 min)
Tuesday	Basic endurance with balance drills and downhill practice (120 min)
Wednesday	Aerobic endurance with 30-min sustained climb at tempo intensity (180 min)
Thursday	Basic endurance with 4 × 30 starting sprint intensities (AC) with 5 min of rest in between (90 min)
Friday	Cross-training, running, or hiking (60-90 min)
Saturday	Basic and aerobic endurance on trails (3 hours)
Sunday	Basic endurance road ride (180 min)

Table 9.7 Weekly Training During the Intense Build or Precompetitive Phase

Monday	Rest or active recovery (30 min)
Tuesday	Aerobic endurance with 6 × 30-sec $\dot{V}O_2$ intensity followed by 5 min at tempo intensity (120 min)
Wednesday	Basic endurance with 60-min climb at aerobic endurance intensity (180 min)
Thursday	Active recovery (45 min)
Friday	Basic endurance with 8 × 90-sec $\dot{V}O_2$ intensity; 3-min recovery (90 min)
Saturday	Trail ride at aerobic endurance to threshold intensity (3 hours)
Sunday	Basic endurance ride with 8 × 15-sec anaerobic capacity sprints with 45 sec of recovery between sprints (120 min)

Ultradistance Cycling Programs

Ultradistance cycling competitions include single-day set-distance races, 24-hour lap races, and multiday and multistage races. The Race Across America (RAAM) is one of the most challenging tests of cycling endurance in the world. It is contested as an individual and team event trying to cover the entire distance (over 3,000 miles, or about 4,830 km) of the continental United States from west coast to east coast. Teams typically take between 6 and 9 days to complete the race, and solo racers finish in 9 to 12 days. Riders sleep very little and average 250 to 350 miles (402-483 km) each day for solo contestants. Other ultradistance events include single-day mountain bike races. Several 3- to 7-day mountain bike stage races are also held around the world, including in South Africa, Costa Rica, the European Alps, and Canadian Rockies. These events are attracting larger crowds each year.

To properly prepare for an ultradistance cycling competition, athletes must have extreme commitment and intelligence in order to avoid overtraining. No one prepares for RAAM by riding from one end of the country to the other before the actual race; therefore, the normal strategy of preparing for a race by doing much more than the actual race itself is not used in the preparation for ultradistance events. Instead, good preparation for ultradistance competitions revolves around building a good endurance base, learning how to pace yourself properly, designing a nutrition and hydration plan that can be implemented on race days, and learning to control the mental difficulties of sleep deprivation and extreme fatigue.

The combination of physical and psychological stresses experienced during ultradistance competitions makes for unpredictable race outcomes. Cyclists must be physically and psychologically prepared for the challenges of ultradistance racing. Tables 9.8 and 9.9 on page 232 provide sample training schedules to be used during the base phase and precompetitive phase for an ultradistance racer preparing for a 24-hour race.

Table 9.8 Weekly Training During the Base or Foundation Phase

Monday	Rest or active recovery (30 min)
Tuesday	Basic endurance (180 min)
Wednesday	Basic endurance with 60-min sustained aerobic endurance intensity (180 min)
Thursday	Active recovery (30 min)
Friday	Cross-training at basic endurance intensity (60 min)
Saturday	Basic and aerobic endurance (6-8 hours)
Sunday	Basic endurance road ride (120 min)

Table 9.9 Weekly Training During the Intense Build or Precompetitive Phase

Monday	Rest or active recovery (30 min)
Tuesday	Aerobic endurance with 3 × 15 min at tempo intensity (150 min)
Wednesday	Basic endurance with 60-min climb at aerobic endurance intensity (180 min)
Thursday	Active recovery (45 min)
Friday	Basic endurance (120 min)
Saturday	Basic and aerobic endurance (6 hours: 3 hours at dusk, 3 hours at night)
Sunday	Basic endurance ride (4 hours)

CHAPTER 10

Swimming

Will Kirousis
Jason Gootman

With the addition of open-water swimming and triathlon to the Olympics, the number of athletes participating in those sports has increased tremendously in recent years. This growth has included athletes of all ages and ability levels, all of whom are excited to improve their endurance swimming abilities. This chapter discusses how to get better at endurance swimming through technique drills, pool-based training, open-water training, and ultradistance training. Because the most common endurance stroke is the front crawl, or freestyle stroke, the drills and training described in this chapter are designed to focus on improving this stroke.

TECHNIQUE DEVELOPMENT

Swimming is a highly technique-dependent sport, more so than most other endurance sports. Technique drills should be a consistent component in an athlete's workouts. The drills at the end of this section can help athletes improve their freestyle technique. With better technique, athletes will achieve the following benefits:

- ▶ **Improved hydrodynamics.** Athletes will move through the water with less resistance, allowing them to move faster and easier.

- ▶ **Efficient pull.** Athletes will be able to generate forward propulsion in the most effective, most powerful way.

- ▶ **More proficiency at swimming in open-water races.** Athletes will be able to navigate the most direct path through the water. They will be able to use the draft of other swimmers. In addition, athletes will be able to cope with the somewhat chaotic nature of swimming in open-water conditions (in ponds, lakes, rivers, or oceans) and swimming with as many as a few thousand other swimmers.

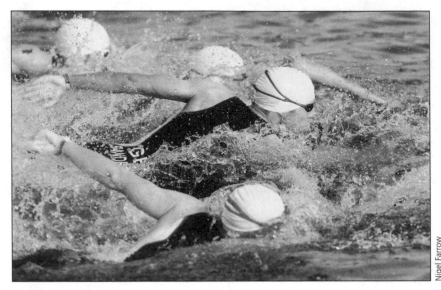

Nigel Farrow

Refining swimming technique improves performance and is vital for open-water swimmers.

The following general guidelines can help swimmers develop good technique in the freestyle:

▶ Swim on the sides, continually rotating from side to side, and spend minimal time flat in the water on the belly. This fosters a long needlelike shape, minimizing drag in the water and increasing hydrodynamics.

▶ Swim high in the water with the hips level with the chest. This helps keep the body in a good horizontal line, preventing the dragging of the hips and legs.

▶ Keep the eyes gazing straight down while swimming the freestyle. This helps maintain a stable point of focus while the body rotates from side to side. It also helps keep the body high in the water by minimizing the disruptions that head movements can cause.

▶ Make sure that the hand enters the water just past the goggles. The hand should effortlessly glide forward as the shoulder and elbow extend naturally with the side rolling. This helps facilitate side swimming, increases hydrodynamics, and fosters the most powerful pull.

▶ Swim with the elbow higher than the hand at all times. The elbow should be kept as high as possible during the pull in order to create the best paddle for pulling the water. During recovery, the elbow should be above the hand so that the arm moves through the shortest, most efficient arc; this conserves energy and helps facilitate side swimming.

▶ Initiate the kick from the hips. Kicking from the hips is the most efficient method. This method improves hydrodynamics by ensuring that the legs trail the body more directly.

Superman

The athlete lies flat on the surface of the water with the arms stretched out like Superman flying through the air. The athlete floats in place with the chest slightly pressed into the water. The athlete should experiment to see how leaning with different amounts of pressure changes the balance. The goal is to be as horizontal as possible—that is, the hips are high in the water, nearly level with the chest.

Vertical Kicking

The athlete is in the deep end of the pool. To start the drill, the athlete allows the body to come to rest vertically, as if treading water with the hands crossed in front of the chest. Instruct the athlete to kick while staying in place and trying to hold the head, neck, and part of the shoulders above the water. The kick should be initiated from the hips, with the knees and ankles bending slightly.

Home Position

The athlete pushes off the wall and rotates so that she is gliding on one side of the body with the top arm at her side and the bottom arm reaching out in front of the body. The chin should be against the bottom shoulder, and the head should be rotated so the eyes are looking straight down at the bottom of the pool. The bottom armpit and ribcage are pressed into the water so that a lift is felt in the body, especially at the hips. The goal is to keep the hips level with the chest. Instruct the athlete to kick smoothly the length of the pool. When the athlete needs to breathe, she should rotate the head only as much as needed to clear the mouth from the water; the athlete should then return the head to the original position.

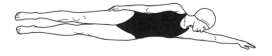

Rotation

The athlete pushes off the wall into the home position. Next, the athlete takes a single stroke with the bottom arm, pausing when the pull is finished, before the recovery starts. The illustrations demonstrate the sequence of actions that the athlete should take during the rotation. The athlete is now in the home position on the opposite side from the start of the drill. The athlete repeats the movement, rotating from side to side and pausing momentarily in the home position on each stroke.

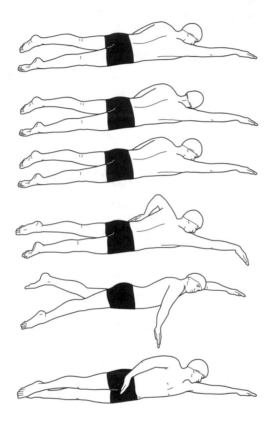

Belly Button

The athlete swims in the normal manner, concentrating on rotating from side to side. Use this cue to help the athlete focus on the rotation: "Point your belly button toward the adjacent lanes or the side walls of the pool."

Downhill

The athlete swims in the normal manner, focusing on slightly pressing the chest into the water as if swimming downhill. Remind the athlete to focus on feeling how the slight pressure keeps the hips high in the water and the body in a horizontal line.

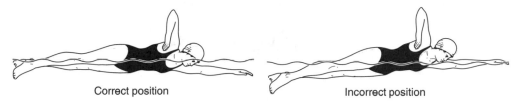

Correct position   Incorrect position

Fingertip Drag

This drill encourages the swimmer to use a relaxed arm recovery. The athlete swims in a normal manner, focusing on dragging the fingertips of the recovery arm across the water during the recovery portion of the stroke. The effectiveness of the drill is enhanced if the athlete maintains a high-elbow position (recovery arm).

Zipper

This drill encourages the swimmer to use a streamlined recovery with minimal excessive motion. The athlete swims normally, focusing on sliding the recovery arm along the side of the body during recovery, as if pulling a zipper up her side. If this is done correctly, the thumb will gently run along the side of the body as the recovery portion of the stroke occurs. As with the fingertip drag drill, the effectiveness of the drill is increased if the athlete maintains a high-elbow position during the recovery.

Barrel

The athlete swims with a normal stroke while pretending to reach over a submerged barrel as the hand enters the water. Emphasis should be on keeping the elbow high and grabbing and holding onto as much water as possible. The illustration shows where the swimmer should imagine the barrel being located. Athletes should not actually attempt swimming over a barrel.

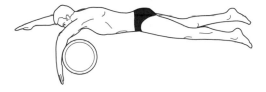

Fist

This drill helps swimmers focus on pulling through the water with the entire forearm. The athlete swims with a normal stroke but closes the hands into fists. This drill can be used as a game by having the athlete try to minimize the number of strokes per length of the pool. The lower the stroke count per length, the more effective the pull.

Catch-Up

This drill helps the swimmer slow down the pulling phase of the stroke, which helps the swimmer maintain horizontal balance. The athlete begins to swim normally but delays each pull until the opposite recovery hand enters the water. The athlete starts in the first position shown in the illustration and then moves sequentially through the remaining positions.

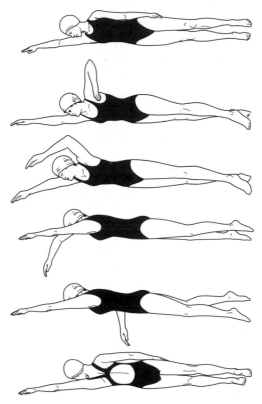

Single-Arm Swim

The emphasis of this drill should be on rotating the body before initiating each pull and on pulling as much water as possible with each stroke. The athlete swims the length of the pool with one arm stroking and the other arm stretched out above the head in front of the body. Breathing should be done to the stroke-arm side. The athlete starts in the first position shown in the illustration and then moves sequentially through the remaining positions.

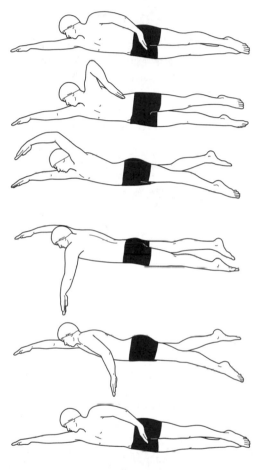

Sighting

This drill is best suited for open-water swimming, and it allows the swimmer to become familiar with swimming in a straight line. The athlete swims, looking up every 8 to 12 strokes to look for the specified sight objects. Make sure the sight objects chosen are large and easily viewed during a quick sight.

Drafting

Learning to draft can allow swimmers to swim at a faster pace and with less energy expenditure than they could alone. This drill requires multiple athletes. Begin the drill with the athletes swimming in a line or in a small group. The goal is for the swimmers behind the lead swimmer to concentrate on staying as close as possible to the toes of the swimmer in front of them. Swimmers should take turns being the lead swimmer.

Contact

This drill is excellent preparation for the contact that is common during open-water swims or the swim segment of a triathlon. This drill requires multiple athletes. The drill begins with the athletes swimming as close as possible to each other. The incidental contact that will occur when the athletes are swimming as close as possible will mimic the contact between swimmers that may occur during open-water competition. Alternate swimmers in the middle of the group so that each athlete learns to experience contact with other swimmers.

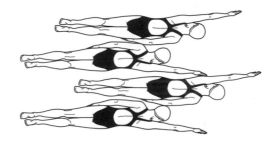

Open-Water Starts

Open-water swims and triathlons may begin on a dock or beach, in shallow water, or in water deep enough to require treading water while waiting for the start of the race. For dock starts, the swimmer should practice diving off a dock and then settling into a good swimming pace as soon as possible. When scouting a location for practicing dock starts, check the depth of the water before diving in headfirst. Depending on the season, water levels near docks may vary, and what initially appears to be deep water can turn out to be shallow on closer examination.

To practice beach starts, the athlete begins on the beach about 15 feet (4.6 m) from the water and sprints into the water until it is not possible to run any farther. At this point, the athlete begins to swim, settling into a good pace as rapidly as possible. To practice shallow-water starts, the athlete should begin in approximately waist-deep water. The athlete dives or falls forward and begins swimming. Finally, to practice deep-water starts, the athlete begins by treading water for about 30 seconds before beginning to swim and settling into a steady swim pace.

Open-Water Swim Exits

This exercise begins with the athlete about 20 yards from land. The athlete swims toward the edge of the water. Once the water depth becomes too shallow for swimming, the athlete stands up and runs toward land, picking the feet up out of the water to reduce the chance of falling.

POOL-BASED TRAINING

Swim distances for this chapter are provided in yards, but the same drills and workouts can be used if athletes are swimming in a meter pool. A well-designed pool-based workout will include the following segments: warm-up (which may include drills), sprint set, main set or sets (commonly called endurance sets), and cool-down. As with all workouts, starting with a good warm-up is important. For pool-based swimming workouts, this is easily accomplished by swimming 200 to 500 yards, building from an easy intensity to an aerobic intensity. In many cases, using a drill set to start a workout serves as a way to simultaneously work on technique and warm up for the more difficult work to come.

Table 10.1 provides five examples of drill sets. Swimmers would perform one of the drill sets at the start of the workout. Because drills are done at a moderate intensity, athletes can perform the drills without any prior warm-up. In this instance,

Table 10.1   Drill Sets

Drill set 1	• Superman: 2 × 30 sec with 10-sec rest interval
	• Vertical kicking: 2 × 30 sec with 10-sec rest interval
	• Single-arm swim: 4 × 25 yards alternating sides with no rest interval
	• 3 × 200 yards as follows (with 10-sec rest intervals):
	  Belly button: 50 yards
	  Fist: 50 yards
	  Downhill: 50 yards
	  Zipper: 50 yards

Drill set 2	• 4 × 150 yards as follows (with 10-sec rest intervals):
	  Rotation: 50 yards
	  Belly button: 50 yards
	  Regular swimming: 50 yards
	• Vertical kicking: 2 × 30 sec with 10-sec rest interval

Drill set 3	• Home position: 4 × 25 yards alternating sides, no rest interval
	• 3 × 250 yards as follows (with 10-sec rest intervals):
	  Fist: 50 yards
	  Zipper: 50 yards
	  Fingertip drag: 50 yards
	  Regular swimming: 100 yards
	• Single-arm swim: 4 × 25 yards alternating sides, no rest interval

Drill set 4	• 3 × 200 yards as follows (with 10-sec rest intervals):
	  Belly button: 50 yards
	  Fist: 50 yards
	  Downhill: 50 yards
	  Zipper: 50 yards
	• Sighting: 200 yards

Drill set 5	• Open-water starts: 4 × each start type (shallow water, treading water, dock, beach) with 30-sec rest intervals • Open-water swim exits: 4 × exit

the purpose of a drill set is to improve or refine technique and to warm up for the rest of the workout. All athletes can benefit from technique work, regardless of current ability level, and using technique work as part of the warm-up process is a very time-efficient method of organizing and executing workouts.

After the warm-up or drill set, sprint sets are an ideal follow-up activity. When sprinting is done early in the workout, the athlete is able to perform each sprint with maximal effort and full energy. Sprinting fosters the development of speed, and all endurance athletes benefit from building and maintaining their speed. Next come the main sets (endurance sets), which are the bulk of an athlete's workout and consist of steady, uninterrupted periods of work or a set of intervals. Finally, the athlete performs a cool-down. The cool-down should consist of about 200 to 500 yards of swimming, decreasing from moderate to low intensity.

As discussed in chapter 2, training zones and terminology need to be defined so that athletes and coaches have a clear understanding of the training expectations. In this chapter, the intensity levels in the workouts are easy (EZ), aerobic (A), anaerobic (AN), and race (R). Swim coaches commonly use these terms to describe intensities. There are no specific parameters for the easy (EZ) intensity. Athletes should simply swim very easy (using an effort level similar to walking).

To determine the other intensity levels, swimmers should use the Swimming 500-Yard Time Trial in chapter 2 (on page 38). The intensity zones for the workouts (excluding EZ) use a percentage range of the time-trial pace as shown in table 10.2. These percentages can then be used to calculate the pace for each intensity level for a specific swimmer based on her time-trial results.

Table 10.2 Determining Swimming Intensity Zones

Intensity zones	Percentage of 500-yard time-trial pace	Heart rate (bpm)
Easy intensity (EZ)	–	–
Aerobic intensity (A)	85-95	77-83
Anaerobic intensity (AN)	95-105	97-103
Race intensity for a sprint-distance triathlon (SDT R)	97-107	98-104
Race intensity for an Olympic-distance triathlon (ODT R)	93.5-105	92-98
Race intensity for a half Ironman (1/2 IM R)	90-100	86-92
Race intensity for an Ironman (IM R)	86.5-96.5	80-86

As an example, if a swimmer completed the 500-yard time trial in 8:00 minutes, the pace per 100 yards is 1:36. This can be calculated in the following manner:

$$\text{Pace per 100 yards} = \text{time} \div 5$$

For the example given, 8:00 minutes divided by 5 equals 1.6 minutes per 100 yards. To convert the .6 into seconds, multiply it by 60 as follows:

$$.6 \times 60 = 36$$

So, the actual pace for the time trial is 1 minute and 36 seconds per 100 yards. Using the percentages for each intensity in table 10.3, the intensity zone ranges can be calculated as follows:

▶ The bottom end of the aerobic intensity zone equals 1:36 ÷ 0.85, or 1:53 per 100 yards. The top end of the aerobic intensity zone equals 1:36 ÷ 0.95, or 1:41 per 100 yards. Thus, the aerobic intensity range equals 1:53 to 1:41 per 100 yards.

▶ The bottom end of the anaerobic intensity zone equals 1:36 ÷ 0.95, or 1:41 per 100 yards. The top end of the anaerobic intensity zone is 1:36 ÷ 1.05, or 1:31 per 100 yards. Thus, the anaerobic intensity range is 1:41 to 1:31 per 100 yards.

The race intensity zone can be calculated in the same fashion. Race intensity only needs to be calculated for the specific race distance of goal races. For convenience, a spreadsheet can be used to calculate intensity zones, and each time a time trial is performed (every 12 to 20 weeks), the intensity zones can be modified as needed.

Using the general workout structure and intensity zones described, coaches and athletes can design numerous pool workouts. Table 10.3 shows several workouts. These workouts can be tailored to meet the needs of individual athletes. Adjust the distances based on the ability levels and goals of the athletes.

Table 10.3 Sample Pool Workouts

Aerobic workout 1	• 4 × 150 yards as follows (with 10-sec rest intervals):
	  Rotation: 50 yards
	  Belly button: 50 yards
	  Regular swimming: 50 yards
	• Vertical kicking: 2 × 30 sec with 10-sec rest interval
	• 6 × 25-yard sprints, going as fast as possible with good form (do the first two at 90% and the rest at 100%)
	• Swim 6 × 300 yards at A intensity with 15-sec rest intervals (rest at the wall for the rest intervals)
	• Cool-down: Swim 300 yards, descending from A to EZ intensity (may use mixed strokes)

Aerobic workout 2	• Home position: 4 × 25 yards, alternating sides, with no rest interval
	• 3 × 250 yards as follows (with 10-sec rest intervals):
	  Fist: 50 yards
	  Zipper: 50 yards
	  Fingertip drag: 50 yards
	  Regular swimming: 100 yards
	• Single-arm swim: 4 × 25 yards, alternating sides, no rest interval
	• 8 × 50-yard sprints, going as fast as possible with good form (do the first two at 90% and the rest at 100%)
	• Swim 600, 500, 400, 300, 200, 100 yards at A intensity with 15-sec rest intervals
	• Cool-down: Swim 300 yards, descending from A to EZ intensity (may use mixed strokes)

(continued)

Table 10.3 Sample Pool Workouts *(continued)*

Aerobic workout 3	• 4 × 150 yards as follows (with 10-sec rest intervals):
	  Rotation: 50 yards
	  Belly button: 50 yards
	  Regular swimming: 50 yards
	• Vertical kicking: 2 × 30 sec with 10-sec rest interval
	• 8 × 50-yard sprints, going as fast as possible with good form (do the first two at 90% and the rest at 100%)
	• Swim 2 × 500 yards at A intensity with 15-sec rest interval
	• Swim 5 × 200 yards at A intensity with 15-sec rest intervals
	• Cool-down: Swim 300 yards, descending from A to EZ intensity (may use mixed strokes)

Anaerobic workout 1	• 3 × 200 yards as follows (with 10-sec rest intervals):
	  Belly button: 50 yards
	  Fist: 50 yards
	  Downhill: 50 yards
	  Zipper: 50 yards
	• Sighting: 200 yards
	• 10 × 25-yard sprints, going as fast as possible with good form (do the first two at 90% and the rest at 100%)
	• Swim 12 × 125 yards at AN intensity with 30-sec rest intervals
	• Cool-down: Swim 300 yards, descending from A to EZ intensity (may use mixed strokes)

Anaerobic workout 2	• Superman: 2 × 30 sec with 10-sec rest interval
	• Vertical kicking: 2 × 30 sec with 10-sec rest interval
	• Single-arm swim: 4 × 25 yards, alternating sides, no rest interval
	• 3 × 200 yards as follows (with 10-sec rest intervals):
	  Belly button: 50 yards
	  Fist: 50 yards
	  Downhill: 50 yards
	  Zipper: 50 yards
	• 10 × 25-yard sprints, going as fast as possible with good form (do the first two at 90% and the rest at 100%)
	• Swim 4 × 300 yards at AN intensity with 30-sec rest intervals
	• Cool-down: Swim 300 yards, descending from A to EZ intensity (may use mixed strokes)

Anaerobic workout 3	• 4 × 150 yards as follows (with 10-sec rest intervals):
	  Rotation: 50 yards
	  Belly button: 50 yards
	  Regular swimming: 50 yards
	• Vertical kicking: 2 × 30 sec with 10-sec rest interval
	• 8 × 50-yard sprints, going as fast as possible with good form (do the first two at 90% and the rest at 100%)
	• Swim 4 × 200 yards at AN intensity with 30-sec rest intervals
	• Swim 8 × 75 yards at AN intensity with 30-sec rest intervals
	• Cool-down: Swim 300 yards, descending from A to EZ intensity (may use mixed strokes)

Long workout 1 (pool)	• Warm-up: Swim 500 yards, building from EZ to A intensity • Swim 5 × 500 yards with 1-min rest intervals (swim the first two at aerobic intensity and the last three at race intensity) • Cool-down: Swim 300 yards, descending from A to EZ intensity (may use mixed strokes)
Long workout 2 (pool)	• Warm-up: Swim 500 yards, building from EZ to A intensity • Swim 2 × 1,000 yards with 1-min rest interval (swim the first one at aerobic intensity and the last one at race intensity) • Cool-down: Swim 300 yards, descending from A to EZ intensity (may use mixed strokes)

OPEN-WATER TRAINING

All endurance swimmers will benefit from open-water training. Specificity is a key component of good training, and because races are in open water, at least some of the swimmer's training should be in open water to allow simulation of race conditions. Open-water swimming is ideal for doing long workouts. Open-water workouts are also a great opportunity to do the technique drills that are best done in open water: sighting, drafting, contact, and buoy turning. A good general framework for an open-water workout could include doing a drill set and then performing a continuous swim; the continuous swim should consist of an aerobic intensity portion and a long-workout portion. Table 10.4 provides several sample open-water workouts.

Table 10.4 Sample Long Open-Water Workouts

Workout 1	• Sighting: 5 min • Drafting: 5 min • Swim 40 min (first 20 min at aerobic intensity, last 20 min at race intensity); throughout the swim, practice the sighting and drafting drills • Back on land, walk for 10 min to cool down
Workout 2	• Open-water starts: 4 × each start type (shallow water, treading water, dock, beach) with 30-sec rest intervals • Open-water swim exits: 4 reps • Swim 1 hour (first 20 min at aerobic intensity, last 40 min at race intensity) • Back on land, walk for 10 min to cool down
Workout 3	• Swim 1 hour (first 20 min at aerobic intensity, last 40 min at race intensity); throughout the swim, practice the contact drill • Back on land, walk for 10 min to cool down

As mentioned, open-water swimming is ideal for long workouts, but other workouts can also be done in open water. For aerobic workouts, athletes swim continuously at an aerobic intensity. Anaerobic workouts need to be less structured than they would be in the pool because there is no pace clock. Fartlek workouts are an excellent option; the athlete swims for a total time or distance with random intervals at anaerobic intensity. Table 10.5 provides sample fartlek-style anaerobic workouts.

Table 10.5 Sample Open-Water Anaerobic Fartlek Workouts

Workout 1	• Swim 1 hour • Start off aerobically, but during the swim include 10 intervals of 1 to 3 min at anaerobic intensity whenever you want to, swimming aerobically after each of them
Workout 2	• Swim 1 hour and 15 min • Start off aerobically, but during the swim include 8 intervals of 3 to 5 min at anaerobic intensity whenever you want to, swimming aerobically after each of them

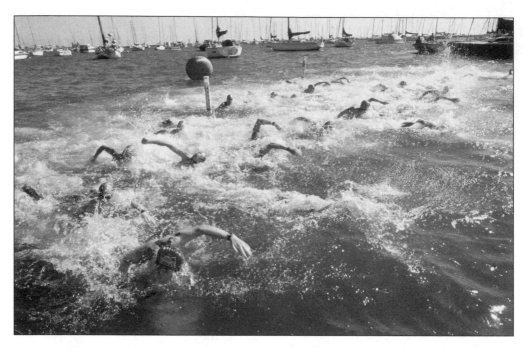

Athletes should prepare for the conditions of an open-water race by training in open water.

Open-water swimming is often performed in cold water. A wetsuit can help improve performance. In very cold conditions, a neoprene swim cap and booties can also be used. If an athlete expects to wear a wetsuit in a race, the athlete should also wear the wetsuit for at least some of the workouts. This will allow the athlete to become familiar with swimming in a wetsuit. Swimming in a wetsuit does provide some flotation, so familiarization is important. Open-water swimming is affected by weather and other natural phenomena such as currents. Within the bounds of safety, athletes should practice swimming in a variety of conditions to ensure well-rounded preparation for their races.

After open-water swims, triathletes can practice swim-to-bike transitions. A mock transition area can be set up, and athletes can swim the final 20 yards, exit the water, and practice transitioning to the bike. If wetsuits will be used in the race, the athlete should also practice wetsuit removal.

USE OF VARIOUS WORKOUTS

Long workouts that include portions at race intensity are the most specific workouts that can be used in training. These workouts should be considered key training sessions. Typically, athletes should do one long workout a week (excluding rest weeks and taper phases). The length of these workouts should increase as the athletes approach their key races. Table 10.6 shows a sample progression of long swims for a triathlete training for an Ironman-length race. The table shows workouts for the 11 weeks before the taper phase for the race.

Long workouts should be done as open-water workouts whenever possible. Pool workouts can be used when the athlete is unable to do an open-water workout.

The remainder of an athlete's workouts each week should be aerobic and anaerobic intensity workouts. Triathletes should typically do two to four swimming workouts a week. Open-water swimmers and ultradistance swimmers should do five or more swimming workouts a week. Triathletes should do one or two anaerobic intensity workouts, one long workout, and the rest as aerobic intensity workouts. Open-water swimmers and ultradistance swimmers should do two or three anaerobic intensity workouts, one long workout, and the rest as aerobic intensity workouts. Aerobic intensity workouts are less stressful than anaerobic intensity workouts, which are more stressful and require more time to recover. The ideal combination of the two intensities provides an athlete with enough workout stress to stimulate improvement while avoiding overtraining.

Table 10.6 Long Swims for a Triathlete Training for an Ironman

Week	Total time (min)	Time at race intensity (min)	Pool alternative
1	30	20	3 × 500 yards, last one at race intensity
2	40	25	4 × 500 yards, last two at race intensity
3	50	30	5 × 500 yards, last three at race intensity
4	Rest week		
5	40	30	4 × 500 yards, last two at race intensity
6	50	35	5 × 500 yards, last three at race intensity
7	60	40	6 × 500 yards, last four at race intensity
8	Rest week		
9	40	35	2 × 1,000 yards, last one at race intensity
10	50	40	3 × 1,000 yards, last two at race intensity
11	60	55	4 × 1,000 yards, last three at race intensity

Table 10.7 provides a guide to the number and type of workouts that should be performed on a weekly basis for certain types of athletes and events. Table 10.8 (on page 249) provides sample workouts based on these recommendations. The workouts presented are for age-group athletes who are beginning to train for these distances. Athletes who are more advanced or skilled may perform more workouts than shown. As mentioned earlier in the chapter, swim training for shorter-distance triathlons will typically be performed a minimum of twice a week (the table indicates three workouts). As the distance of the event increases, so do the number of workouts; this number may increase to as many as 10 to 12 for a high-level ultradistance swimmer.

In general, all triathlon training should include one long swim. Shorter-distance triathlon training would include two additional workouts—one at aerobic intensity and the second at anaerobic intensity. At higher performance levels and longer distances, no more than two additional anaerobic intensity workouts would be performed, and the remaining workouts would be done at aerobic intensity. The triathlete needs to balance the demands of swimming with the demands of running and cycling training. Chapter 11 of this book provides information on how to balance training for the multiple events.

Table 10.7 Weekly Number and Types of Workouts for Various Athletes

Type of swimmer or event	Number and type of workouts
Sprint	3 workouts per week • 1 long workout • 1 aerobic intensity • 1 anaerobic intensity
Olympic	3-4 workouts per week • 1 long workout • 1-2 aerobic intensity • 1 anaerobic intensity
Ironman	3-4 workouts per week • 1 long workout • 1-2 aerobic intensity • 1 anaerobic intensity
Ultradistance swimmer	5 or more workouts per week* • 1 long workout • 2 aerobic intensity • 2 anaerobic intensity

*Additional workouts should include no more than 1 additional workout at AN intensity, and the remainder should be at A intensity.

Table 10.8 Sample Training Weeks for Triathletes (Non-Elite) and Open-Water Swimmers

Type of swimmer or event			
Sprint triathlon	**Olympic triathlon**	**Ironman triathlon**	**Open-water or ultradistance swimmer***
Long workout			

Pool
• Warm-up: Swim 500 yards, building from EZ to A intensity
• Swim 1 × 1,000 yards
• Cool-down: Swim 200 yards easy
Total: 1,700 yards
	Pool
	• Warm-up: Swim 500 yards, building from EZ to A intensity
	• Swim 2 × 1,000 yards with 1-min rest interval
	  First at aerobic intensity
	  Last at race intensity
	• Cool-down: Swim 300 yards easy
	Total: 2,800 yards
		Open water
		• Open-water starts: 4 × each start types (shallow water, treading water, dock, and beach) with 30-sec rest intervals
		• Open-water race exits: 4 reps
		• Swim 1 hour
		  First 20 min at aerobic intensity
		  Last 40 min at race intensity
		• Back on land, walk 10 min to cool down
			Open water
			• Sighting: 5 min
			• Drafting: 5 min
			• Swim 40 min
			  First 20 min at aerobic intensity
			  Last 20 min at race intensity
			  Throughout the swim, practice the sighting and drafting drills
			• Back on land, walk 10 min to cool down

Aerobic intensity workout 1			

Pool
• 3 × 150 yards as follows (10-sec rest intervals):
  Rotation: 50 yards
  Belly button: 50 yards
  Regular swimming: 50 yards
• Vertical kicking: 2 × 30 sec with 10-sec rest interval
• 4 × 25-yard sprints, going as fast as possible with good form; do the first two at 90% and the rest at 100%.
• Swim 2 × 300 yards at A intensity with 15-sec rest interval (rest at the wall)
• Cool-down: Swim 150 yards, descending from A to EZ intensity (may use mixed strokes)
Total: 1,300 yards
	Pool
	• 4 × 150 yards as follows (10-sec rest intervals):
	  Rotation: 50 yards
	  Belly button: 50 yards
	  Regular swimming: 50 yards
	• Vertical kicking: 2 × 30 sec with 10-sec rest interval
	• 4 × 25-yard sprints, going as fast as possible with good form; do the first two at 90% and the rest at 100%.
	• Swim 3 × 300 yards at A intensity with 15-sec rest intervals (rest at the wall)
	• Cool-down: Swim 200 yards, descending from A to EZ intensity (may use mixed strokes)
	Total: 1,800 yards
		Pool
		• 4 × 150 yards as follows (with 10-sec rest intervals):
		  Rotation: 50 yards
		  Belly button: 50 yards
		  Regular swimming: 50 yards
		• Vertical kicking: 2 × 30 sec with 10-sec rest interval
		• 6 × 25-yard sprints, going as fast as possible with good form; do the first two at 90% and the rest at 100%.
		• Swim 6 × 300 yards at A intensity with 15-sec rest intervals (rest at the wall)
		• Cool-down: Swim 300 yards, descending from A to EZ intensity (may use mixed strokes)
		Total: 2,850 yards
			Pool
			• 4 × 150 yards as follows (with 10-sec rest intervals):
			  Rotation: 50 yards
			  Belly button: 50 yards
			  Regular swimming: 50 yards
			• Vertical kicking: 2 × 30 sec with 10-sec rest interval
			• 8 × 50-yard sprints, going as fast as possible with good form; do the first two at 90% and the rest at 100%.
			• Swim 2 × 500 yards at A intensity with 15-sec rest interval
			• Swim 5 × 200 yards at A intensity with 15-sec rest intervals
			• Cool-down: Swim 300 yards, descending from A to EZ intensity (may use mixed strokes)
			Total: 3,300 yards

*5+ workouts/week

(continued)

Table 10.8 Sample Training Weeks for Triathletes (Non-Elite) and Open-Water Swimmers (*continued*)

Type of swimmer or event			
Sprint triathlon	Olympic triathlon	Ironman triathlon	Open-water or ultradistance swimmer*
Aerobic intensity workout 2			

		Pool
		• 4 × 150 yards as follows (with 10-sec rest intervals):
		  Rotation: 50 yards
		  Belly button: 50 yards
		  Regular swimming: 50 yards
		• Vertical kicking: 2 × 30 sec with 10-sec rest interval
		• 6 × 50-yard sprints, going as fast as possible with good form; do the first two at 90% and the rest at 100%.
		• Swim 2 × 400 yards at A intensity with 15-sec rest interval
		• Swim 4 × 200 yards at A intensity with 15-sec rest interval
		• Cool-down: Swim 200 yards, descending from A to EZ intensity (may use mixed strokes)
		Total: 2,700 yards
			Pool
			• Home position: 4 × 25 yards, alternating sides, no rest interval
			• 3 × 250 yards as follows (10-sec rest intervals):
			  Fist: 50 yards
			  Zipper: 50 yards
			  Fingertip drag: 50 yards
			  Regular swimming: 100 yards
			• Single-arm swim: 4 × 25 yards, alternating sides, no rest interval
			• 8 × 50-yard sprints, going as fast as possible with good form; do the first two at 90% and the rest at 100%.
			• Swim 600, 500, 400, 300, 200, 100 yards at A intensity with 15-sec rest intervals
			Total: 3,450 yards

*5+ workouts/week

			Type of swimmer or event
			Open-water or ultradistance swimmer*
Sprint triathlon	**Olympic triathlon**	**Ironman triathlon**	
Anaerobic intensity workout 1			

Pool
• 3 × 150 yards as follows (10-sec rest intervals):
  Rotation: 50 yards
  Belly button: 50 yards
  Regular swimming: 50 yards
• Vertical kicking: 2 × 30 sec with 10-sec rest interval
• 4 × 50-yard sprints, going as fast as possible with good form; do the first two at 90% and the rest at 100%.
• Swim 3 × 150 yards at AN intensity with 30-sec rest intervals
• Swim 4 × 75 yards at AN intensity with 30-sec rest intervals
• Cool-down: Swim 200 yards, descending from A to EZ intensity (may use mixed strokes)
Total: 1,600 yards
	Pool
	• 4 × 150 yards as follows (10-sec rest intervals):
	  Rotation: 50 yards
	  Belly button: 50 yards
	  Regular swimming: 50 yards
	• Vertical kicking: 2 × 30 sec with 10-sec rest interval
	• 4 × 50-yard sprints, going as fast as possible with good form; do the first two at 90% and the rest at 100%.
	• Swim 4 × 150 yards at AN intensity with 30-sec rest intervals
	• Swim 6 × 75 yards at AN intensity with 30-sec rest intervals
	• Cool-down: Swim 200 yards, descending from A to EZ intensity (may use mixed strokes)
	Total: 2,050 yards
		Pool
		• Superman: 2 × 30 sec with 10-sec rest interval
		• Vertical kicking: 2 × 30 sec with 10-sec rest interval
		• Single-arm swim: 4 × 25 yards, alternating sides, no rest interval
		• 3 × 200 yards as follows (10-sec rest intervals):
		  Belly button: 50 yards
		  Fist: 50 yards
		  Downhill: 50 yards
		  Zipper: 50 yards
		• 10 × 25-yard sprints, going as fast as possible with good form; do the first two at 90% and the rest at 100%.
		• Swim 4 × 300 yards at AN intensity with 30-sec rest intervals
		• Cool-down: Swim 300 yards, descending from A to EZ intensity (may use mixed strokes)
		Total: 2,450 yards
			Pool or open water
			• Swim 1 hour
			• Start off aerobically, but during the swim include 10 intervals of 1 to 3 min at anaerobic intensity whenever you want to, swimming aerobically after each of them

Anaerobic intensity workout 2			
			Pool or open water • Swim 1 hour and 15 min • Start off aerobically, but during the swim include 8 intervals of 3 to 5 min at anaerobic intensity whenever you want to, swimming aerobically after each of them

*5+ workouts/week

ULTRADISTANCE TRAINING

Athletes training for ultradistance swims must consider some other training factors in addition to those discussed previously. Because the races can be as long as 10 miles or more, training must focus on developing a high level of endurance.

Here are some key training factors for ultradistance swimmers:

1. To successfully complete an ultradistance swim, athletes need to use a high training volume.
2. Achieving a high training volume requires a high training frequency. Athletes may need to complete swims twice a day for most days of the training week.
3. Athletes should use long workouts that will specifically prepare them for racing. For example, a swimmer training for a five-mile swim should perform long workouts that build up to that distance.

Table 10.9 shows a sample progression of long swims. This table shows the long workouts for the 11 weeks before the taper phase for the race. All of these long workouts should be done at approximately race intensity, which will be aerobic intensity or slightly lower.

Table 10.9   Sample Progression of Long Swims for an Ultradistance Swimmer

Week	Total time
1	1 hour
2	1 hour and 30 min
3	2 hours
4	Rest week
5	1 hour and 30 min
6	2 hours
7	2 hours and 30 min
8	Rest week
9	2 hours
10	2 hours and 30 min
11	3 hours

CHAPTER 11

Triathlon

Denny DePriest

Triathlon distances range from the sprint distance to the ultradistance. Sprint-distance triathlons include any triathlon with a distance less than the international distance. The international distance for triathlons, more commonly known as the Olympic distance, consists of a 1,500-meter (.9 mile) swim, 40 kilometers (24.8 miles) of cycling, and 10 kilometers (6.2 miles) of running. This distance provides many nonexperienced triathletes with an opportunity to compete in the sport. With the distances being relatively short, the average triathlon participant can complete these races in around 2.5 to just over 3 hours. Triathletes at the professional elite level generally complete the distances in just less than 2 hours. For the nonprofessional elite athlete, the Olympic distance is also appealing because the training volume required is not as overwhelming (as discussed later in the chapter).

The half-Ironman triathlon is composed of 1.9 kilometers (1.2 miles) of swimming, 90 kilometers (56 miles) of cycling, and 21 kilometers (13.1 miles) of running. This distance is very appealing to athletes who want to challenge themselves after they have a few international-distance triathlons under their belt. The swim is only slightly longer, while the bike and run offer more of an endurance challenge.

Besides the Olympic gold medal, the title of Ironman champion is the most sought-after reward in triathlon. The Ironman distance is composed of 3.9 kilometers (2.4 miles) of swimming, 180 kilometers (112 miles) of cycling, and 42 kilometers (26.2 miles) of running. The original Ironman triathlon was held in Hawaii, and this distance is now raced on every corner of the globe. The Ironman World Championships are held every year in October on the weekend of the full moon. Slots in this competition are awarded to top professional and age-group athletes. The Ironman triathlon involves great physiological demands and requires a great time commitment from those who plan to participate.

Most triathletes are age-group athletes who get involved in the sport for various reasons. Many are runners, cyclists, or swimmers who have suffered an injury and embark on triathlon as a form of cross-training. Other age-group athletes are looking for new challenges beyond their current health and fitness hobbies. In triathlon, age groups are separated by 4 years. Most triathlons include age categories beginning at 18 to 21 and going up in 4-year increments. Participants are usually required to compete in the appropriate age group based on their age on December 31 of the present year.

Elite triathletes are often athletes who have had great success in one of the three disciplines at the collegiate level. Those professional triathletes who did not come from a collegiate swimming or running background sometimes find it difficult to compete on the International Triathlon Union (ITU) stage. These elite athletes are generally more successful at the longer-distance events. Though the ITU format is a draft-legal format for the cycling phase, many people do not recognize the excellent swimming and running performances that occur in these events. They view the draft-legal format as a nonpure triathlon. This is simply not true considering the pace that participants swim and run at these races. Many times the men swim the 1,500 meters in under 17 minutes or slightly above, while the best women in the world run the 10 kilometers in around 34 minutes (3:24 per kilometer pace).

TRAINING TIME REQUIREMENTS

The amount of time required for triathlon training will depend on the distance the athlete is pursuing and the goals of the athlete. Athletes should also take into account their personal time requirements, such as family, social life, and work. The sprint and international distances offer opportunities that require much less training time. Athletes can also race these distances multiple times per year without the fear of overreaching and overtraining. Races at these distances are common, and most athletes will have a number of races to choose from in their area. In many states, such as North Carolina, a series of races are held that present athletes with the opportunity to compete nearly every month of the spring and summer (sometimes even several times in a month). As long as an athlete is not overracing, this is a great and fun opportunity. It also provides some motivation for the athlete to get in some aerobic endurance work during the winter months.

Training requirements for the sprint-distance triathlon can be as few as 8 hours per week. For the international-distance triathlon, athletes can often train effectively using an average of 10 hours per week. Of course, some ITU athletes normally train 20 to 30 hours per week, and they put in 15 to 18 hours of training during their recovery weeks. For the half-Ironman and Ironman distances, the time commitments required are substantial. Having family and other support networks is important for athletes who compete at these distances. These events require longer training weeks, and most triathletes who work will spend a lot of time on weekends performing longer rides and runs. In addition, the time required to recover from these training events often interferes with social engagements.

When deciding which distance to pursue, athletes must first determine their personal goals. Then they need to determine why they are competing in the sport. These steps often allow athletes to make smart decisions before they choose an event that becomes too time consuming later on down the road. Athletes must always remember that the sport should be fun and enjoyable. Triathlon training is one of the healthiest lifestyles that a person can choose to participate in. First-time triathletes often register for distances far greater than their present abilities. This can lead to potential injury and undue stress—physiological, social, and emotional stress. Athletes must set realistic goals and must be honest with themselves.

Many charitable organizations offer training groups and coaches that will help an athlete get started in triathlon with international-distance events. This is a great way to start in the sport, but athletes must be leery of the distances that are beyond their experience level, even if the events are for a good cause. If athletes train smart and safe, their race day will be enjoyable and safe as well. Athletes who are unsure of which distance to choose should always start with a local sprint triathlon. After the race, these athletes will feel good about their accomplishment and will also be able to gauge whether they need a few more sprints before embarking on events that cover greater distances. Just because an athlete has completed a number of marathons does not mean that the athlete is ready for the Ironman.

TRANSITIONS

Regardless of the distance of the triathlon, the transitions from one discipline to the next are an essential part of every race and an important part of training. T1 is the transition from the swim to the bike, and T2 is the transition from the bike to the run. Both transitions are unique and require a different approach for success. Athletes should practice everything during training and should not attempt new things during race day.

On T1, when exiting the water, the athlete's main priority is vision. If wearing a wetsuit, the athlete needs to get the wetsuit down to slightly below the hips. On arriving at the bike, the athlete should get the suit down as far as possible toward the ankles and step out of the suit; the athlete should stow the suit in the transition bin or at least out of the way of other athletes (not in another athlete's transition area).

Novice triathletes commonly transition from the swim to the bike without their shoes already attached to the pedals. Having the shoes attached to the pedals can speed up the transition time, but the athlete needs to work on this during training. To work on this skill, athletes can leave their shoes attached to the pedals, and on every training ride, they will need to get in and out of the shoes as they begin or conclude the ride. Indoor trainer sessions offer an excellent opportunity to practice. Using rubber bands, attach the heel of the shoe to some part of the bike. Water cages and rear skewers are both excellent attachment points. The shoes should be attached to the bike so that the athlete begins the ride with the shoes parallel to the ground; this allows the athlete to mount the bike and get moving as quickly as possible. Once the athlete has gotten her speed up, she can put one foot in the shoe. The athlete can make tension adjustments (with the straps of the shoes) after both feet are in the shoes.

On T2, athletes should end the ride the same way they began by getting their feet out of the shoes in a similar manner. About 200 meters (or yards) away from the bike transition, the athlete can take one foot out and regain race speed. The athlete then takes the second foot out and has both feet on top of the shoes until he is ready to dismount. Once the athlete gets to the dismount line, the athlete gets off the bike; the athlete can travel with the bike by placing one hand on the seat or using the stem. The stem is preferred because of the many mishaps that can happen on the way to the transition area. If racing at a venue that offers a flow-through transition area, which is common in ITU events, athletes should also ensure that they are on the same side that their bike rack is on before getting to the dismount line. This saves time and prevents the athlete from having to cross over the flow-through area.

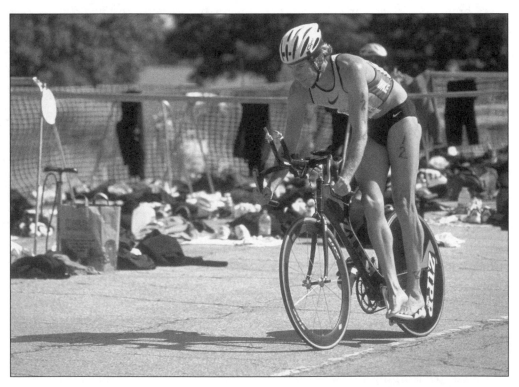

Practicing how to transition helps athletes move smoothly through a triathlon.

Once the athlete gets to her bike rack, she places the bike in the rack to the best of her ability using either the handlebars, seat, or rear tire. The rack type will dictate which method is preferred. Once the bike is racked, the athlete removes her helmet and puts her running shoes on. Many athletes will use elastic laces in their shoes that allow them to slip on the shoes very quickly. When the athlete begins running out of the T2 area, a good strategy is to begin running with a very short and quick cadence. The legs need to get used to running off the bike. When the athlete takes shorter and quicker strides, this allows the neuromuscular system to aid in getting the athlete into a normal running stride after a few hundred meters. The athlete can then settle in and run at race pace. In elite races, quick transitions offer an opportunity for athletes to surge ahead and create a gap between them and their competition.

RACE PREPARATIONS

Athletes need to complete a race prep once they arrive at the local area of the competition. Reconnoitering the course itself is a great benefit. For longer events, driving the bike course is a great way to learn the course and become familiar with any turns, hazards, and feeding areas. In most longer-distance events, a "special needs" area is set up where athletes can place items in a bag that will be handed to them during the race. For shorter events, athletes can ride the course itself if they arrive at the venue a few days early. Athletes should walk both transition areas and visualize themselves in the race. They should locate the bike rack areas, changing tents, and anything that is unique to the venue and may not be common at every race. Knowing where they will be running to and from will help athletes visualize their success on race day and will lower the stress caused by fear of the unknown. Race prep workouts should be short in duration; athletes will not gain any fitness in the week of the race.

Swimming sections of the course is also a good idea. Athletes should identify what they will be using for sighting markers on race day. They can also become familiar with the currents as well as the entrance and exit points. They should take note of things such as how deep the water is at the entrance and exit, or what the bottom surface is like (smooth, rocky, and so on). Knowing these things allows the athlete to be more confident and develop a race day strategy.

On race day, athletes often feel anxious and nervous. They should realize that this is normal and have some positive self-talk phrases to help them relax. Nutrition is very important, and the athlete shouldn't change anything from training. Athletes should focus on getting a good night's sleep the second day out from the race. Most race start times are very early, and with the prerace nervousness, the night before is not the best night to count on getting a lot of sleep.

On race day, athletes should conduct the warm-up that they planned with their coach. The bike warm-up should be performed first so that there is time to deal with any maintenance issues. The athlete should take the bike out for an easy quick ride, going through all of the gears and conducting a few accelerations. On returning to the T1 area, the athlete should do one last look-over, check the bolts one last time, and add a little lube on the chain. At this point, the athlete should know that the bike is ready to go. Athletes should leave their bike in the gear that they want to start the ride in; that way, the athletes will not be doing a lot of gear changing while trying to get into their shoes. Next, the athlete should head out for a quick run, running the same path she will follow to exit after the bike phase of the race. This is one last chance to check the surface and look for any potential hazards. The athlete should keep the run very short and then return to T2. The athlete then puts on her wetsuit or just grabs her cap and goggles (if not using a wetsuit for the race) and heads out for a quick warm-up swim and return. Then the athlete should be ready to go for her wave start time or the mass-start time. A good practice is for athletes to keep a water bottle with them as they wait for their start. They can dispose of the bottle just before the race start.

DURING THE RACE

When the race begins, athletes should do what they have been doing in training to prepare for the race. They should not get out of rhythm or deviate from their race plan. Less experienced athletes are often advised to start to the side and in the back to avoid some of the chaos that is associated with swim starts. This should depend on the athlete's training. If the athlete is confident in his swimming ability, he should not be afraid to mix it up a little and put himself in a good position. Moreover, for less experienced swimmers, "off to the side" may also mean a longer distance. Athletes should just do what they have done in training and be honest with themselves about their abilities. Most athletes are very nervous before the swim start. The biggest error that can be made here is going out too hard at the start of the swim.

During the swim, the athlete needs to realize that contact is part of the sport. Many athletes get frustrated with this portion of the race. Being kicked or hit is common. Athletes should not let this take them out of their focus and rhythm. They should remain calm and focus on moving away from or in front of the person. Swimmers are not intentionally making contact with others, so if contact occurs, an athlete should not take it personally. Making turns around buoys can sometimes be very frustrating. Athletes should just focus on getting around it and moving on. Everyone has to make the turn, and in a mass start, it is very chaotic. Knowing this going in, athletes can mentally go through this challenge and focus on staying calm and relaxed.

When exiting the swim and proceeding to T1, athletes should go through the same things that they did in practice and get to their bike. The athlete gets his wetsuit and other swim gear off, puts his helmet on, and heads out on the bike. The athlete should start hydrating right away. If the athlete had a bad swim, he should put it behind him and refocus on his cycling effort. Using a heart rate monitor or power meter is an excellent way for athletes to stay at the proper intensity on race day. Athletes should ride within their abilities, which they should know from their

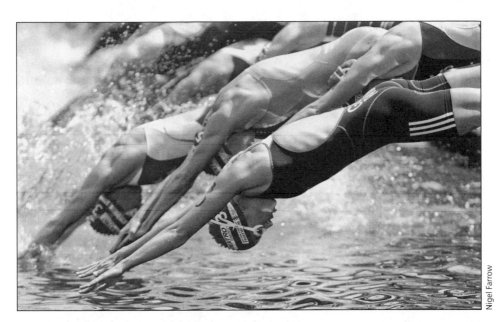

Nigel Farrow

At the beginning of a race, triathletes should focus on their race plan to calm their nerves and set their pace.

training rides. If an athlete has a mechanical problem or flat tire, he must not let it stress him out to the point of losing focus. There is nothing he can do about it. The athlete needs to think positive and do what must be done to get back in the race. During the bike segment, the athlete should make a conscious effort to maintain proper hydration and nutrition. Athletes must remember that what they eat and drink on the bike sets up their running ability. To help ensure that their race day plan is carried out as intended, athletes can use a timer on their watch or write their plan on a piece of tape and mount it on their top tube.

Heading into T2, the athlete should begin to visualize the transition, remembering where his bike rack is located (or what side his bike rack is on for flow-through transition areas). The athlete dismounts just before the dismount line and begins heading to the transition point. The athlete racks his bike, takes his helmet off, puts on his running shoes, and begins running. The athlete should keep the cadence short and quick (as described earlier) and should execute the transition the same way as in training. As the run progresses, the athlete needs to keep his pace and intensity within his limitations, remember to carry out his hydration and nutrition plan, and finish out the race strong.

After finishing a race, athletes should begin the recovery process immediately. Hydration and nutrition are essential. Athletes will have plenty of time to analyze their performance later. They should get a massage if possible and continue to focus on recovery. After the race has been over for a couple of hours or days, the athletes can then analyze their performance. They should take pride in their accomplishments and make notes about what they can do differently next time. This will allow the athletes to address some key components for future training.

TRIATHLON PROGRAM DESIGN

Triathlon is a single sport made up of the activities of running, biking, and swimming. Like sports that involve only one of these activities, triathlon training is optimized when the training program is periodized. The same principles of periodization that were discussed in previous chapters also hold true for triathlon training programs. The coach or athlete needs to keep in mind that balancing training for all three activities makes triathlon program design more complicated than the design for single-activity sports. However, the periodization of training is essential for maximizing performance and enjoyment of the sport.

It is always a good idea for an athlete to work with a certified coach throughout the process. The coach can offer sound advice and help figure out scheduling conflicts that are common among athletes. Understanding periodization models while balancing personal and professional life can be very challenging. Athletes who are venturing into the self-coached world need to have as many resources as possible.

For many amateur athletes, training programs follow an annual plan that is usually developed at the end of a previous competitive or training year. For example, in the northeastern part of the United States, the annual plan is typically developed in the late fall. The annual plan is divided into training periods, or macrocyles. For some elite athletes, such as a runner with Olympic team aspirations, the training plan may be designed to cover a 4-year period rather than an annual period. As noted in earlier chapters, the macrocycle typically refers to the largest training period. For most athletes, this is the annual training plan that is created at the end of each season for the following season. The annual plan is divided into large phases called macrocycles, which can be as long as 3 months.

A mesocycle is a shorter period within the macrocycle. For triathlon training, each mesocycle should have a primary focus of improving aerobic endurance, strength endurance, or power endurance and can be discipline specific. Microcycles are smaller training phases within the mesocycle. These generally continue for a 7- to 10-day period. For each microcycle plan, a volume and volume of intensity (VOI) are specified for each discipline within each workout. Every workout will include a warm-up, a main set or prescribed VOI, and a cool-down. The VOI in swimming is commonly referred to as the main set of the workout. For cycling, this would include the intervals at which the athlete will repeat hills or hold a specific wattage or cadence. For running, this may include intervals that include distance and time at the track, timed intervals on a hill, or specific cadence turnover rates. Some of the running workouts use a Rating of Perceived Exertion (RPE) scale from 6 to 20, where a 6 would be an easy effort and a 20 a maximal effort. The VOI can be manipulated in work-to-rest ratios to target specific energy systems in the aerobic and anaerobic development of each individual athlete.

Each training phase includes a primary focus. For base periods, the primary focus is aerobic endurance. Build periods have an emphasis on race-specific demands that may include anaerobic endurance or any skills that need to be addressed during training. Precompetition periods involve fine-tuning and allow the athlete to maintain intensity while reducing volume; these periods conclude with a race taper designed to help the athlete achieve a peak performance in the race. Athletes who are training for their first event may not be aiming to achieve their highest level of performance; however, finishing the race within a certain time or just covering the distance still requires the body to be rested and ready on race day.

TRAINING PLANS

This section provides some sample weekly training plans for each distance in triathlon. Remember that one size does not fit all. These are only samples that will help athletes and coaches understand how to create training plans. For all the workouts described, the speed, intensity, or wattages may be modified based on the training intensity protocols for an individual athlete. For cycling sessions, some of the described workouts require a power device; athletes who do not have the required device can modify the workouts and train based on heart rate (either outdoors or inside on a stationary trainer).

Figures 11.1 (on page 262), 11.2 (on page 264), and 11.3 (on page 266) provide sample weekly training plans for the base, build, and precompetition phases for a beginning triathlete training for a sprint-distance triathlon. Notice that the training programs include resistance training sessions, as well as increasing levels of intensity and volume from the base to build phases. For the precompetition phase, volume is reduced in conjunction with a further increase in intensity to allow preparation for the intensities of racing. Athletes who are participating in triathlon training for enjoyment—and not for competition—may not need to use such strict periodization. A significant reduction in volume occurs during the precompetition phase. For the athlete who is training for health and enjoyment, this reduction in training time may not be desired. Reduced training volume is essential for those athletes seeking to train for optimal performance.

Figures 11.4 (on page 268), 11.5 (on page 270), and 11.6 (on page 272) provide sample weekly training plans for the base, build, and precompetition phases for an elite athlete competing in Olympic-distance triathlons. As with the sprint training, the plans include an increase in volume and intensity from base to build phases, followed by increased intensity and reduced volume during the precompetition phase. Notice the inclusion of trail running for part of the running program. As the triathlon distances increase, so does the training volume. A greater volume will increase the potential chance for injuries. Performing trail running for part of the run training will reduce the impact for some of the running work. Trails are a much softer surface than roads or sidewalks. Many successful triathletes train on soft surfaces for the majority of their training to help reduce the risk of developing training injuries.

Figure 11.1   Base Week for a Sprint-Distance Triathlon

MONDAY

Swim	Run
Warm-up • 200 m choice • 6 × 50 m (25 m drill, 25 m free) on 1:00-1:10 • 2 × 100 m (25 m free, 50 m nonfree, 25 m free) on 2:00-2:10 Main set (VOI 500 m) • 100, 300, 100 m on 1:50 Cool-down • 200 m easy pull, 200 m easy mixed stroke Total: 1,400 m	Run and walk (walk 5 min, run 10 min) at an easy aerobic effort • RPE: 12 • Athlete should be able to maintain a conversation with a training partner Repeat the walk-run combo for a total of 30 min

TUESDAY

Bike	Run
Spin class	Easy aerobic run for 20 min

WEDNESDAY

Swim	Resistance
Warm-up • 200 m free, 200 m choice • 10 × 50 m (25 m drill choice, 25 m free) Main set (VOI: 600 m) • 100, 200, 100, 200 m with 20-sec rest intervals • Record times and average your pace per 100 m Cool-down • 300 m choice Total: 1,800 m	2 × 15 straight-leg deadlift with barbell (if possible) 2 × 15 stability ball wall squat with arms out in front 2 × 10 stability ball push-up 2 × 10 stability ball crunch 2 × 10 stability ball back extension

THURSDAY

Bike	Run
Spin class	Repeat Monday's run with these changes: • Add 30 sec to the run portion • Deduct 30 sec from the walk portion

FRIDAY

Swim	Resistance
Warm-up • 300 m choice (200 m as 50 m free, 25 m drill, 25 m free, 50 m nonfree, 50 m free) • 10 × 50 m Odd reps are 25 m kick, 25 m free Even reps are 25 m drill, 25 m free All with 15-sec rest intervals Main set (VOI: 1,000 m) • 2 × 100 m with 20-sec rest intervals • 2 × 400 m, trying to maintain the average pace from Wednesday; 20-sec rest intervals Cool-down • 200 m choice Total: 2,000 m	4 × 10 (each leg) single-leg stability ball squat 3 × 30 sec push-up holding position on stability ball Superset • 3 sets of the following: 30 sec sit-up extension with legs out and back flat 20 sec elbow push-up position on stability ball 2 × 30 stability ball crunch 2 × 30 stability ball back extension

SATURDAY

Bike	Run
45-60 min ride • Keep effort aerobic • Do not exceed RPE 12	Easy aerobic run for 25 min

SUNDAY

Rest day for all disciplines

Figure 11.2 Build Week for a Sprint-Distance Triathlon

MONDAY

Swim	Run	Resistance
Warm-up • 1 × 300 m (50 m free with pull buoy, 50 m backstroke × 3) Main set • 1 × 400 m pull (25 m catch-up, 25 m catch-up with foot drag, 50 m tempo free × 4) • 1 × 300 m kick (25 m kick right side, 25 m kick left side, 25 m free, 25 m 6 kick 1 stroke, 25 m 6 kick 3 stroke, 25 m free × 2) • 1 × 800 m (25 m of each IM stroke) If you have problems with any of the four strokes, replace the stroke with 25 m of choice, preferably free • 4 × 75 m sprints with descending rest intervals 45 sec, 30 sec, 15 sec Cool-down • 1 × 200 m Total: 2,300 m	20-35 min of easy running • Keep effort at an easy aerobic pace; RPE 12	3 × 10 stability ball reverse hyperextension 3 × 10 (in each direction) stability ball weighted twist (you may choose to use no weight) 2 × 10 stability ball ab roller 2 × 10 stability ball reverse ab roller 2 × 20 sec stability ball table 2 × 10 wall bangers

TUESDAY

Bike for 1 hour after completing a 10-min easy spin warm-up. Ride a rolling course with 5-8 climbs of 1-2 min in duration. Work on staying seated during the climb.

WEDNESDAY

Swim	Run
Warm-up • 1 × 300 m (100 m free, 50 m drill choice × 2) Main set • 1 × 500 m free; rest 45 sec with pull buoy • 1 × 400 m free; rest 45 sec • 1 × 300 m free; rest 30 sec with pull buoy • 1 × 400 m free; rest 45 sec • 1 × 500 m free; rest 45 sec with pull buoy Cool-down • 1 × 100 m Total: 2,500 m	Run easy for 10 min to warm up. Run 4 × 3 min at race effort with 2 min of recovery running in between. After the last 2-min recovery run, walk for 5 min to cool down.

THURSDAY

Bike	Resistance
Spin class	2 × 10 stability ball push-up with hands on the ball 2 × 10 stability ball hyper hug 2 × 10 stability ball lateral raise 2 × 5 stability ball pass 5-point touches 1 round right leg, left arm 1 round left leg, right arm 1 round right leg, right arm 1 round left leg, left arm 2 × 12 wall bangers

FRIDAY

Rest day for all disciplines

SATURDAY

Swim	Bike	Run
Warm-up • 1 × 300 m Main set • 4 × 50 m sprints with 30-sec rest intervals • 1 × 500 m free; rest 45 sec with pull buoy • 1 × 400 m free; rest 45 sec • 1 × 300 m free; rest 30 sec with pull buoy • 1 × 400 m free; rest 45 sec • 1 × 500 m free; rest 45 sec with pull buoy and paddles Cool-down • 1 × 100 m Total: 2,700 m	Bike for 1.5 hours • Ride 30 min to warm up • For the next 45 min, ride 6 min in your aerobars and 3 min in your drops or brake hoods • Ride the last 15 min easy	Run off the bike for 15 min • Run 3 min at race pace, then 2 min of recovery running for 3 rounds to equal the 15 min

SUNDAY

30-40 min easy walk and stretch

Figure 11.3   Precompetition Week for a Sprint-Distance Triathlon

MONDAY

Swim	Run
Warm-up • 1 × 300 m choice • 10 × 50 m build on 1:00 Main set • 1 × 200 m on 1:40-1:50 and sighting last 100 m • 1 × 400 m on 1:40-1:50 and sighting last 100 m Cool-down • 1 × 300 m (50 m free, 100 m back, 50 m free, 100 m choice) Total: 1,700 m Volume of intensity: 600 m • Adjust intervals as needed	20-min run • 10 min of easy running to warm up • 5 min of 20 sec at race pace, 40 sec easy • Run the last 5 min easy

TUESDAY

Bike	Run
Ride for 45-60 min • 4 × 3 min at race effort in aerobars with 2-min easy spin recoveries • Ride easy for remaining time	Run off the bike for 10 min at easy aerobic effort

WEDNESDAY

Rest day for all disciplines

THURSDAY

Swim	Bike
Warm-up • 1 × 300 m choice (50 m free, 25 m kick, 25 m free) on 1:40 On first 25 m kick, kick on side with no arm extended on the right side On second 25 m kick, kick on side with barrel roll On third 25 m kick, kick on side with no arm extended on the left side • 5 × 50 m build on 1:00 Main set • 3 × 100 m, 3 × 50 m (focus on head position and turnover on the 50s; sight at race speed on the last 25 m of the 100s) 100s on 1:50-2:00 50s on 0:50-0:55 Cool-down • 1 × 200 m choice Total: 1,200 m Volume of intensity: 450 m	Spin class right after swim

FRIDAY

Bike	Run
Ride easy for 20-30 min with 30-sec race efforts at 10-, 12-, and 14-min points • Clean your bike, check all bolts, and lube the chain • Go through your prerace checklist for all equipment	Warm up for 5 min. Then perform an easy 20-min run with a 15-, 30-, and 45-sec pickup to race pace; recovery interval should be twice the amount of time of the pickup.

SATURDAY

Race day

SUNDAY

Rest day for all disciplines

Figure 11.4 Base Week for an Olympic-Distance Triathlon (Elite)

MONDAY

Swim	Run	Resistance
Swim with masters team	15-min easy aerobic endurance run before your strength and conditioning session	Leg press: descending sets of 15, 12, 10, 8 Deadlift: descending sets of 15, 12, 10, 8 Single-leg extension: descending sets of 10, 8 Leg curl: descending sets of 10, 8 2 × 10 (each leg) side lunge 2 × 15 stability ball back extension Hold in the up position for 5 sec

TUESDAY

Bike for 90 min at an easy aerobic endurance effort. Stay in the small chain ring. Effort should not exceed an RPE of 12.

WEDNESDAY

Swim	Run

Warm-up
• 300 m free, 100 m nonfree, 100 m free
• 10 × 100 m (25 m free, 25 m kick, 25 m drill, 25 m free on 1:00-1:10)
• 4 × 50 m building pace throughout on 1:00
Main set
• 8 × 100 m, 1 × 800 m
   Hold 100 m pace + 2 sec per 100 for the 800 m
• 2 × 400 m
   1 with fins, 2 with paddles; both easy aerobic effort
Cool-down
• 200 m choice easy
Total: 4,300 m
Volume of intensity: 2,400 m
	45-min trail run
	• Count foot strikes every 3 min for 15 sec. Your goal is 23 right-foot or left-foot strikes. This will give you a turnover of 92 foot strikes per min.

THURSDAY

Bike	Resistance
90-min ride • Keep effort easy; RPE 12 • During the first 20 min of the ride, conduct spin-ups for 30 sec (building by 10 sec) at the 6-, 12-, and 18-min points. • During the last 5 min, practice getting in and out of your cycling shoes several times	Dumbbell bench press: descending sets of 12, 10, 8, 6 Single-arm dumbbell row: descending sets of 12, 10, 8, 6 3 × 10 rear deltoid raise 3 × 10 hammer curl 3 × 10 single-arm triceps extension Stability ball back extension: descending sets of 20, 15, 10 1 × 12 stability ball pass

FRIDAY

Swim	Run
Warm-up • 1 × 300 m choice • 5 × 100 m (25 m kick, 25 m free, 25 m drill, 25 m free) • 5 × 100 m (25 m kick on side with head down and no lead hand, 25 m free × 2) • 10 × 50 m (25 min max) 3 plus strokes on second 25 m Main set • 4 × 200 m descending on 1:25-1:30 • 4 × 250 m On odd reps, pull with paddles; on even reps, no paddles; on 1:30-1:40 Cool-down • 400 m choice • Adjust send-offs as needed Total: 4,000 m Volume of intensity: 1,800 m	1-hour fartlek run

SATURDAY

Bike	Run
Ride for 2-2.5 hours on rolling terrain • Keep effort aerobic; stay seated on all climbs	Run for 45-50 min off the bike • Keep effort aerobic

SUNDAY

Run	Resistance
1:15-1:30 run • Keep effort aerobic	Yoga class

Figure 11.5 Build Week for an Olympic-Distance Triathlon (Elite)

MONDAY

Swim	Bike	Resistance
Warm-up • 300 m choice; take HR • 5 × 100 m (25 m SAR*, 25 m free, 25 m SAL**, 25 m free) on 1:40 • 10 × 50 m on 55 (first 10 strokes fist, the rest free) • 5 × 100 m building pace after the first 50 m on 1:30-1:40 Main set • 2 × 100, 200, 300, 200, 100 m on 1:20 • 4 × 200 m pull with paddles on 2:50 Total: 4,400 m Volume of intensity: 2,600 m	90-min easy spin, small chain ring only • Conduct this workout later in the day after your strength and conditioning session.	Leg press: descending sets of 15, 12, 6 3 × 10 leg extension 3 × 10 leg curl 3 × 10 (each leg) side lunge

*SAR=single arm right (swim only with the right arm)
**SAL=single arm left (swim only with the left arm)

TUESDAY

Swim	Bike	Run
3K active recovery: choice	2-hour bike with aerobic climbing 3 × 3K climbing seated with standing for the last 500 m.	45-min easy aerobic endurance run

WEDNESDAY

Swim	Run

Warm-up
• 1 × 600 m free
• 10 × 100 m (25 m kick with barrel roll, 25 m free, 25 m drill, 25 m free) with 10-sec rest intervals
• 5 × 100 m on 1:25-1:30 (one 25 m focus point and one 25 m free)
  Focus points: 1. head position, 2. catch, 3. pull, 4. rotation, 5. recovery
Main set
• 5 × 100 m on 1:15
• 2 × 500 m descend by 100 on 120-130
• 5 × 100 m based on 500 m time plus 5 sec for send-off
• 2 × 250 m with sighting in last 50 m (10-sec rest interval)
Total: 4,600 m
Volume of intensity: 2,500 m
	Track session
	• 10-min easy run to warm up
	• Dynamic warm-up with running drills
	Main set
	• 3 × 2K at 3:06-3:09 per K pace
	  Rest 90 sec between repeats
	• 3 × 1K at 3:00-3:03 per K pace
	  Rest 2 min between the 1K repeats
	• Cool down with 10 min of barefoot running on the grass
	• Ice and massage after this workout

THURSDAY

Bike	Run	Resistance
2-hour aerobic endurance ride • Work on cornering in and out of turns without braking. Accelerate out of turns for 10-15 sec (in and out of the saddle for the accelerations).	45-min aerobic endurance run • Conduct this run later in the day	Dumbbell incline bench press: descending sets of 15, 12, 6 Standing straight-arm lat pull-down: descending sets of 15, 12, 6 2 × 15 lateral deltoid raise 2 × 15 straight bar curl 2 × 15 rope triceps extension 3 × 20 stability ball back extension 2 × 8-10 stability ball push-up

FRIDAY

Swim	Bike
Warm-up • 1 × 400 m (100 m free, 100 m back, 100 m free, 100 m choice) • 6 × 100 m (25 m drill, 25 m free × 2 on 1:30-1:40) • 1 × 500 m descend by 100 on 1:30-1:40 Focus points for 100s: 1. head position, 2. catch, 3. pull, 4. rotation with finish, 5. recovery Main set • 2 × (4 × 50 m build by 25, 1 × 200 m with sighting, 2 × 50 m first 25 high turnover) on 1:20-1:30 Rest 1 min between rounds • 1 × 500 m (100 m back, 100 m choice, 25 m kick, 25 m free × 2) • Adjust send-offs as needed Total: 3,000 m Volume of intensity: 1,500 m	90-min active recovery ride (small chain ring)

SATURDAY

Swim	Bike	Run
Swim 5K with masters or university team Volume of intensity for main set should be within 2,500-3,000 m	CompuTrainer: ride for 5 min to calibrate; ride 5 more min easy building to 225 watts Main set • Round 1: 3 min at 275 watts 2 min at 400 watts 1 min easy at <200 watts 4 min at 300 watts 90 sec at 425 watts 2 min easy at <200 watts 5 min at 350 watts 1 min easy 30 sec at 450 watts 3 min easy • Round 2: 5 × 45 sec building by 25 watts per 15 sec beginning at 425 watts up to 475 watts (with 3 min easy <200 watts) Cool-down • Spin down for 10 min after run at 100 watts	2 × 2K off the bike • On the treadmill, goal is 3:10-3:12 per K pace • 90 sec in between repeats • IT band stretches and walk for recovery

SUNDAY

90-min aerobic endurance run

Figure 11.6 Precompetition Week for an Olympic-Distance Triathlon (Elite)

MONDAY

Swim	Bike
Warm-up: 1,500 m Main set • 2 rounds of 10 × 50 m under 35 sec on 50 m send-off; 1 min between rounds Cool-down: 500 m Total: 3,000 m Volume of intensity: 1,000 m	CompuTrainer: 1-hour bike Warm up for 15 min Main set • 3 × 5 min at 325, 350, 375 watts, with 5-min recoveries • 2nd round: 3 × 1 min building by 20 at 425, 450, 475 watts, with 3-min recoveries Cool down for 5 min

TUESDAY

Swim	Bike	Run
Warm-up • 1 × 400 m (100 m free, 100 m back, 100 m free, 100 m choice) • 5 × 100 m (25 m drill, 25 m free × 2) on 1:30-1:40 • 1 × 500 m descend by 100 on 1:30-1:40 Focus points for 100s: 1. head position, 2. catch, 3. pull, 4. rotation with finish, 5. recovery Main set • 2 × (4 × 75 m build by 25 m, 1 × 100 m with sighting, 2 × 50 m first 25 sprint) on 1:20-1:30 Rest 1 min between rounds • 1 × 300 m (100 m back, 100 m choice, 100 m back) Total: 2,700 m Volume of intensity: 1,300 m • Adjust intervals as needed	Early-morning 1-hour ride; wash, lube, clean, and pack bike	Treadmill Warm up for 5 min Main set • Run at race pace for 2, 4, 2, 4, 2, 4, 2 min, with 50% of the interval time for recovery • Cool down for 5 min

WEDNESDAY

Travel day

Swim	Bike	Run
If a swim is possible, swim 1,500 m choice; RPE of 10-12	Once you have arrived, assemble your bike and ride easy for 10-15 min. Go through all of the gears. Tighten all bolts and lube the chain once you have returned.	If no swim option is available, run easy for 10-15 min and stretch. Include dynamic flexibility and running drills as part of the run.

THURSDAY

Swim	Bike	Run
Warm-up • 1 × 300 m choice • 10 × 50 m build on 1:00 • 3 × 100 m IM on 1:30-1:40 Main set • 1 × 200 m, 4 × 50 m, 400 m sighting last 100 m of 200 and 400 m on 1:20-1:30 • 1 × 300 m (50 m free, 100 m back, 50 m free, 100 m choice) Total: 2,200 m Volume of intensity: 1,100 m • Adjust intervals as needed	Bike easy 30-45 min • Ride 1-2 loops of the course • Sit on climbs after 15-sec jump to initiate simulated attack halfway up • Work on gearing to know what gear you need to be in to push over the top • Ride easy for 5-10 min back to hotel	Run easy for 20-25 min Main set • After 10 min of running, conduct 15-, 30-, and 45-sec pickups to 3-5 sec faster than race pace per K with 2 times the volume for recovery • Run easy for remaining time

FRIDAY

Swim	Bike
Open-water practice on course • 3 starts and reentries • Adjust intervals Total: 1.5-2K Volume of intensity: 3-5 × 30 sec of race efforts	Ride course • 15-sec jump on top of 3rd climb with work over the top • Only 1 loop today • Preview T1 and T2 with estimated start number

SATURDAY

Swim	Bike	Run
Easy 20-min swim with 2-3 race accelerations around buoys and off of a pontoon • Practice at least 1 exit and reentry • Walk through T1 as recovery and remove wetsuit at estimated rack number	On flat section of course, ride 2 × 30, 1 × 1 min efforts • Work drops with first 15 sec standing out of saddle, good rhythm • No climbs today; go out and back on flat bottom section • Rehearse getting in and out of shoes at appropriate place • Go through mental scenarios that may take place during the race	Run 15-20 min • Go through prerace warm-up • Easy run in and out of T2 with 3 × 30 sec pickups to race pace

SUNDAY

Race day

Beginning triathletes who are transitioning into Olympic-distance triathlons should keep in mind that these sample programs may contain a higher volume and intensity level than they are prepared to undertake. A beginning triathlete with the goal of completing an Olympic-distance triathlon should be able to successfully complete each of the event distances before beginning to consider a higher training volume. The sample programs are excellent templates, but experience and athletic ability (as well as life responsibilities—job, family, and so on) play a role in determining the level of training that an athlete is able to undertake.

Figures 11.7, 11.8 (on page 277), and 11.9 (on page 278) provide sample weekly training plans for the base, build, and precompetition phases for athletes training for a half-Ironman triathlon. Figures 11.10 (on page 279), 11.11 (on page 281), and 11.12 (on page 283) provide similarly phased plans for athletes training for an Ironman triathlon. Both of these sample training programs are designed for a non-elite athlete, but they are intended for an athlete with a level of experience significantly higher than a beginner. All athletes, even experienced athletes, should seek the advice of an endurance coach when developing a training plan for these longer-distance events.

As indicated in the training programs, training for a half-Ironman or Ironman triathlon requires a serious time commitment. Notice that the Ironman training program doesn't simply double the training volume of a half-Ironman program. The increased training volumes for races of this distance means that athletes need to be very careful to ensure that injuries do not occur, especially during the running training. More training does not always equal better performance. Many endurance coaches know that the most difficult thing about working with half-Ironman and Ironman athletes is making sure they don't do too much training without enough rest and recovery.

Many successful triathletes never compete in races longer than sprint or Olympic distances. The longer distances, in addition to taking more training time, also require a much higher skill set for success. Most athletes can train for 3 to 4 months and successfully complete a sprint triathlon. However, being able to bike 56 miles and then run a half marathon takes a significant level of fitness that may take a number of annual plans to develop.

Figure 11.7 Base Week for a Half-Ironman Triathlon

MONDAY

Bike	Run
90-min ride on stationary trainer • Ride for 20 min to warm up • For next 10 min, conduct ILT drills as 20 sec right leg, 20 sec both legs, 20 sec left leg at the 2-, 4-, 6-, and 8-min points • Ride for remaining time at an easy aerobic effort	1-hour run with hills • Keep effort aerobic • On hills, focus on pulling the arms back to drive the knee higher in order to maintain stride length • Do not push the effort on the downhills and flats

TUESDAY

Resistance	Swim	Run

Complete this band routine before swim session
• 2 sets with 1 min between sets. Sets are continuous between exercises.
  10 double-arm pulls
  10 triceps extensions
  10 front raises
  10 single-arm side raises
  10 chest presses
  10 single-arm pulls
• Alternate as in swimming (moderate to fast)
  10 internal rotator
  10 external rotator
  10 sit-ups
• Handles at shoulders and anchor point behind you
	Warm-up
	• 1 × 300 m choice
	• 10 × 50 m (25 m drill, 25 m free)
	• 10 × 50 m (25 m kick on side with head down and no lead hand, 25 m free)
	• 10 × 50 m (25 m one-arm stroke right hand out front, 25 m left hand out front)
	  Simulate going around buoys
	Main set
	• 3 × 300 m
	  Descend beginning on 1:35 base for round 1
	  1:30 base for round 2
	  1:25 base for round 3
	• 2 × 500 m with fins and snorkel
	  Focus on head position on 1:30-1:35
	• Adjust send-offs as needed
	Total: 3,700 m
	Volume of intensity: 1,900 m
		45-min aerobic endurance run
		• Count your right-foot or left-foot strikes for 15 min every 5 min. Your goal is 22-23 foot strikes per 15 sec.

WEDNESDAY

90-min trainer ride. After a 20-min warm-up, ride 10 × 3-min intervals. On odd intervals, use an undergear cadence of 100-110 rpm. On the even intervals, use an overgear cadence of 65-75 rpm. Conduct all intervals with a 2-min recovery period of easy spinning. Ride easy for the remaining time.

(continued)

Figure 11.7 Base Week for a Half-Ironman Triathlon *(continued)*

THURSDAY

Swim	Run	Resistance
Masters swim practice Total: 5K Volume of intensity: 1,800-2,200 m	30-min aerobic endurance run just after your swim	Leg press: descending sets of 25, 20, 15 3 × 20 double-leg extension 3 × 20 leg curl 3 × 15 (each leg as lead) walking lunge 2 × 30 stability ball back extension Make this the last workout of the day just before dinner

FRIDAY

Swim	Bike
3K aerobic endurance (choice)	1-hour easy aerobic endurance spin; keep cadence above 95 rpm for the duration

SATURDAY

Bike	Run
4-hour aerobic endurance ride • Warm up for 20-30 min • Ride for 3.5 hours at 10-15 bpm below your LT	Run off the bike for 1 hour at aerobic endurance effort • Record average pace and heart rate • Stay on flat to rolling terrain

SUNDAY

Swim	Resistance
3K active recovery swim with long continuous sets • Work on lengthening your stroke and efficiency • Do this later in the day a few hours after your run; RPE <10	Run 90-105 min at RPE 12-14

Figure 11.8 Build Week for a Half-Ironman Triathlon

MONDAY

Swim	Resistance
Masters swim practice Total: 5K Volume of intensity: 1,500-1,800 m	Dumbbell single-arm bench press: descending sets of 25, 23, 20 Dumbbell single-arm row: descending sets of 25, 23, 20 2 × 20 rear deltoid raise 2 × 20 hammer curl 2 × 20 single-arm triceps extension Stability ball back extension: descending sets of 25, 20

TUESDAY

Rest day for all disciplines

WEDNESDAY

Swim	Resistance
Masters swim practice Total: 5K Volume of intensity: 2,200-2,500 m	Leg press: descending sets of 25, 20, 15 3 × 20 double-leg extension 3 × 20 leg curl 3 × 15 (each leg as lead) walking lunge 2 × 30 stability ball back extension

THURSDAY

Rest day for all disciplines

FRIDAY

Masters swim practice (5K total volume; VOI of 2,500-2,800 m)

SATURDAY

Bike	Run
2-hour bike ride • Bike to the hill loop, ride 2 times up and over, then ride back easy If cancelled because of weather, ride easy for 30 min on a CompuTrainer; for the hill repeat section, ride the CompuTrainer Richer pass course, and then ride in aero position for remaining time.	Run off the bike on trail, road, or treadmill for 1 hour at half-marathon pace

SUNDAY

Swim	Run
2K active recovery swim with long continuous sets • Work on lengthening your stroke and efficiency • Do this later in the day a few hours after your run; RPE <10	90-min aerobic endurance run with 6 × 8 min at race pace minus 5 sec per mile (all with 4-min recoveries)

Figure 11.9 Precompetition Week for a Half-Ironman Triathlon

MONDAY

Swim	Bike
Masters swim practice Total: 3K Volume of intensity: 1,000-1,500 m	90-min bike • Easy aerobic effort (RPE 12) with 4 × 5-min race efforts with 5-min recoveries • Spin easy for remaining time

TUESDAY

Bike	Run
60-min bike • Aerobic endurance spin with spin-ups for 30-45 sec building by 15 sec every 10 min • Clean and pack your bike for travel	45-min run with 15-, 30-, and 45-sec efforts up to 10K effort (with recovery time of 3 times the duration of the effort) • Focus on form and cadence (22-23 foot strikes per 15 sec)

WEDNESDAY

Travel day. Once you arrive at the race location and are settled in, assemble your bike and take it out for a quick spin to ensure there are no issues. If your flight or drive is long, remember to walk around during the flight or when stopping to refill your vehicle with gas. In addition, muscular activation can be done while seated. If the flight is longer than 4 hours, compression socks are highly recommended.

THURSDAY

Swim	Bike
Nice and easy swim on swim course • Get a feel for the swim start area • Swim easy with some long efficient stroke work • Include some backstroke just to stretch out from the travel	Ride for 45-60 min • Easy aerobic ride; just stretch out your legs from travel

FRIDAY

Swim	Bike	Run
Swim at the course • Practice sighting, entries, and exits; notice any obstacles and landmarks • Conduct 3-5 hard efforts with long recoveries • Focus on long efficient strokes • Walk through T1 and find out where your bike will be for tomorrow's race	45-min ride • Ride to T2 and first 5 miles of the bike course with spin-ups for 20 sec every 8 min • Check your bike one last time before bike turn-in	15-min easy run and stretch

SATURDAY

Race day

SUNDAY

Rest day for all disciplines

Figure 11.10 Base Week for an Ironman Triathlon

MONDAY

Swim	Resistance
Warm-up • 1 × 300 m (100 m free, 50 m drill choice × 2) • 1 × 500 m free; rest 45 sec with pull buoy • 4 × 200 m free; rest 30 sec with paddles • 2 × 300 m free; rest 30 sec with pull buoy and paddles • 2 × 400 m free; rest 30 sec with paddles • 1 × 500 m free; rest 30 sec with pull buoy and paddles Cool-down: 1 × 100 m Total volume: 3,600 m	Dumbbell incline bench press: descending sets of 15, 12, 10 Standing straight-arm lat pulldown: descending sets of 15, 12, 10 Lateral deltoid raise: descending sets of 15, 12, 10 Straight bar curl: descending sets of 15, 12, 10 Rope triceps extension: descending sets of 15, 12, 10 5 × 10-12 stability ball back extension 2 × 10-12 stability ball push crunch

TUESDAY

Bike	Run

Warm-up
• Ride for 5 min and calibrate the CompuTrainer in the stand-alone mode
• Ride for 10 more min easy (not to exceed zone 2 HR)
  At the 4-, 6-, and 8-min points, conduct 3 × 30-sec spin-ups building your cadence each 10 sec
  During the 3rd 10 sec, when you begin to bounce in the saddle, come back down to a cadence that you can maintain without bouncing
Main set
• 6 × 5 min at 210 watts with 5 min of recovery between 130-140 watts
  During the 5 min, add 15 watts every min to increase an additional 75 watts by the end of the 5-min work interval
Cool-down: 12 min
• During the cool-down, conduct 5 × 1 min of ILT work with 20 sec right foot, 20 sec both feet, and 20 sec left foot
• Cool down for the remaining time with easy spinning at 100-125 watts
	45-min run with tempo intervals
	• Warm up with easy running and running drills
	• Conduct 4 × 3 min sets building your effort throughout. The efforts should have a quick turnover and a slight increase in respiration.
	• Each interval should be followed by a 2-min easy recovery run
	Cool down with easy running and stretching

(continued)

Figure 11.10 Base Week for an Ironman Triathlon *(continued)*

WEDNESDAY

Swim	Resistance
Swim with masters group	Leg press: descending sets of 15, 12, 10 3 × 15 double-leg extension 3 × 15 leg curl 3 × 10 walking lunge 3 × 15-20 stability ball back extension

THURSDAY

Bike	Run
2-hour aerobic endurance ride (small chain ring only)	45-min easy aerobic endurance run; keep effort in zone 2 or aerobic endurance

FRIDAY

Swim	Run
Warm-up • 1 × 600 m drill (50 m free, 25 m fist, 50 m free, 25 m × 3, 25 m free, 25 m fist, 100 m free) • 10 × 50 m building pace by 25 m on 1:00 Main set • 3 × 200 m with 30-sec rest interval • 10 × 50 m (all under 45 sec on 1:10) • 1 × 200 m freestyle by 100 m; good solid efforts Cool-down • 1 × 300 m (choice) Total: 2,700 m Volume of intensity: 1,300 m	1-hour run on rolling terrain • Maintain an aerobic endurance effort not to exceed RPE 12 • If you exceed RPE 12 on hills, walk to bring the intensity back down

SATURDAY

Bike	Run
3-hour ride with long gradual climbs of 6-8% in grade • Attempt to stay seated throughout the climbs • Use climbs of at least 4-6 min in duration	Run off the bike easy for 40 min

SUNDAY

Run	Resistance
2.5-hour aerobic endurance run; RPE 12-13 • Run on trails or grass	3 × 10 stability ball reverse hyperextension 3 × 10 stability ball weighted twist in each direction (you may choose to use no weight) 2 × 10 stability ball ab roller 2 × 10 stability ball reverse ab roller 2 × 20 sec stability ball table 2 × 10 wall banger

Figure 11.11   Build Week for an Ironman Triathlon

MONDAY

Swim	Bike	Resistance

Warm-up
• 300 m choice, free, drill
  Rest for 45-60 sec
Main set
• 40-min continuous swim
• Count your strokes every 100 m during the last 25 min
  Attempt to keep them consistent
Cool-down
• 200 m with 100 m of LA combo (4 backstroke, 3 free) and 100 m of super slow free
	1:15-1:30 ride on flat to rolling roads
	• Keep effort at aerobic level
	• Stay seated on all climbs
		Yoga class

TUESDAY

Swim	Bike

Swim with masters group	Warm-up
	• Ride for 5 min and calibrate the CompuTrainer in the stand-alone mode
	• Ride for 10 more min easy (not to exceed zone 2 HR)
	  At the 4-, 6-, and 8-min points, conduct 3 × 30-sec spin-ups building your cadence each 10 sec
	  During the 3rd 10 sec, when you begin to bounce in the saddle, come back down to a cadence that you can maintain without bouncing
	Main set
	• 6 × 4 min at 250-270 watts with 4 min of recovery at 125-150 watts
	  During the 4 min, add 15 watts every min to increase an additional 60 watts by the end of the 4-min work interval
	Cool-down
	• For 12 min, conduct 5 × 1 min of ILT work with 20 sec right foot, 20 sec both feet, and 20 sec left foot
	• Cool down for the remaining time with easy spinning at 100-125 watts

(continued)

Figure 11.11 Build Week for an Ironman Triathlon *(continued)*

WEDNESDAY

Two runs for 1:15 each. First run is before work, and second run is after work. During both runs, maintain your pace at 8:00 to 8:10 minutes per mile. Use heart rate zone 2 for both runs.

THURSDAY

Swim	Bike	Resistance
Swim with masters group	Recovery ride: relax and focus on the mechanics of the pedal stroke; maintain a cadence of 95-100 rpm • Stay within zone 1 for the entire length of the ride • Do not exceed the beginning of your zone 2 for this ride • For the entire ride, stay in the small chain ring and focus on bringing the knees in over top of the pedals	Pilates class

FRIDAY

Rest day for all disciplines

SATURDAY

6-hour bike ride. Warm up for 20-30 min. Then ride 5.5 hours at your race effort. Hydrate and eat as planned for race day. Keep effort at an aerobic endurance effort but work the hills with some standing climbs.

SUNDAY

Bike	Run
Ride for 4 hours on rolling to hilly terrain	Run off the bike for 60 min at half-marathon effort

Figure 11.12 Precompetition Week for an Ironman Triathlon

MONDAY

Swim	Run
Warm-up • 300 m choice, free, and drill Main set • 30-min continuous swim counting your strokes every 100 m during the last 25 min Attempt to keep them consistent Cool-down • 200 m with 100 m of LA combo (4 backstrokes, 3 free) and 100 m of super slow free	Warm-up including 4-5 pickups Then 4 × 90 sec (recover 3 min) at half-marathon pace

TUESDAY

Bike 1 hour easy on flat to rolling hills. Conduct 6-8 spin-ups at preferred cadence plus 10 for 20 sec. Ride easy for the last 10-15 min. On completion, clean and pack your bike.

WEDNESDAY

Travel day. Once you arrive at the race location and are settled in, assemble your bike and take it out for a quick spin to ensure that there are no issues. If your flight or drive is long, remember to walk around during the flight or when stopping to refill your vehicle with gas. Also, muscular activation can be done while seated. If the flight is longer than 4 hours, compression socks are highly recommended.

THURSDAY

Swim	Run
Swim nice and easy on the swim course. • Get a feel for the swim start area, and so forth. • Swim easy with some long efficient stroke work. Some backstroke is also included to stretch out from travel.	Easy aerobic run for 20-30 min • Use the start and finish of the course • Note landmarks • Include several accelerations to race pace • Otherwise, keep heart rate in zone 1

FRIDAY

Swim	Bike
Open-water practice on course Total: 1.5-2K Volume of intensity: 3-5 × 30 sec of race efforts • Work on sighting for landmarks • Walk through swim exit to T1 in order to feel comfortable for tomorrow's race	Ride for 45-60 min • Ride easy aerobic effort with 3-4 spin-ups to preferred cadence plus 10 • Start and end the ride in T1 exit and T2 entrance points • Cool down on the way back to your hotel • Clean, lube, and check all bolts before bike turn-in tonight

SATURDAY

Race day

SUNDAY

Active recovery in all disciplines

References

Chapter 1

Astrand, P-O., K. Rodahl, H.A. Dahl, and S.B. Stromme. 2003. *Textbook of work physiology*. Champaign, IL: Human Kinetics.

Brooks, G.A., T.D. Fahey, and K.M. Baldwin. 2005. *Exercise physiology: Human bioenergetics and its application*. New York: McGraw-Hill.

Hoffman, J. 2002. *Physiological aspects of sport training and performance*. Champaign, IL: Human Kinetics.

Marieb, E.N., and K. Hoehn. 2006. *Human anatomy and physiology*. Redwood City, CA: Benjamin/Cummings.

McArdle, W.D., F.I. Katch, and V.L. Katch. 2006. *Exercise physiology: Energy, nutrition and human performance*. Philadelphia, PA: Lippincott, Williams and Wilkins.

Moore, K.L., and A.F. Dalley. 2005. *Clinically oriented anatomy*. Philadelphia, PA: Lippincott, Williams and Wilkins.

Mougios, V. 2006. *Exercise biochemistry*. Champaign, IL: Human Kinetics.

Sharkey, B.J., and S.E. Gaskill. 2006. *Sport physiology for coaches*. Champaign, IL: Human Kinetics.

Wilmore, J.H., D.L. Costill, and W.L. Kenney. 2007. *Physiology of sport and exercise*. Champaign, IL: Human Kinetics.

Chapter 2

Brooks, G., T. Fahey, and K. Baldwin. 2004. *Exercise physiology: Human bioenergetics and its applications*. 4th ed. Columbus, OH: McGraw-Hill.

Gore, C. (Ed.) 2004. *Physiological tests for elite athletes*. Champaign, IL: Human Kinetics.

Hoffman, J. 2002. *Physiological aspects of sport training and performance*. Champaign, IL: Human Kinetics.

Janssen, P. 2001. *Lactate threshold training*. Champaign, IL: Human Kinetics.

Maud, P., and C. Foster. (Eds.) 2006. *Physiological assessment of human fitness*. 2nd ed. Champaign, IL: Human Kinetics.

McArdle, W., F. Katch, and V. Katch. 2006. *Exercise physiology: Energy, nutrition, and human performance*. 6th ed. Baltimore, MD: Lippincott Wilkins and Williams.

Weltman, A. 1995. *The blood lactate response to exercise*. Champaign, IL: Human Kinetics.

Chapter 3

Bompa, T. 1999. *Periodization: Theory and methodology of training*. Champaign, IL: Human Kinetics.

Bompa, T., and M. Carrerra. 2005. *Periodization training for sports*. Champaign, IL: Human Kinetics.

Chaouachi, A., C. Castagna, M. Chtara, M. Brughelli, O. Turk, O. Galy, K. Chamari, and D.G. Behm. 2010. Effect of warm-ups involving static or dynamic stretching on agility, sprinting, and jumping performance in trained individuals. *The Journal of Strength and Conditioning Research* 24(8): 2001-2011.

Kentta, G., and P. Hassmen. 1998. Overtraining and recovery: A conceptual model. *Sports Medicine* 26(1): 1-16.

Mujika, I., and S. Padilla. 2003. Scientific bases for precompetition tapering strategies. *Medicine and Science in Sports and Exercise* 35(7): 1182-1187.

Pyne, D.B., I. Mujika, and T. Reilly. 2009. Peaking for optimal performance: Research limitations and future directions. *Journal of Sports Science* 27(3): 195-202.

Zaryski, C., and D.J. Smith. 2005. Training principles and issues for ultra-endurance athletes. *Current Sports Medicine Reports* 4(3): 165-170.

Chapter 4

Armstrong, L.E., D.J. Casa, M. Millard-Stafford, D.S. Moran, S.W. Pyne, and W.O. Roberts. 2007. American College of Sports Medicine position stand. Exertional heat illness during training and competition. *Medicine and Science in Sports and Exercise* 39(3): 556-572.

Australian Institute of Sport. www.ausport.gov.au/.

Bernadot, D. 2006. *Advanced sports nutrition.* Champaign, IL: Human Kinetics.

Castellani, J.W., A.J. Young, M.B. Ducharme, G.G. Giesbrecht, E. Glickman, and R.E. Sallis. 2006. American College of Sports Medicine position stand. Prevention of cold injuries during exercise. *Medicine and Science in Sports and Exercise* 38(11): 2012-2029.

Coleman, E. 2003. *Eating for endurance.* Boulder, CO: Bull Publishing.

Gerard-Eberle, S. 2007. *Endurance sports nutrition.* Champaign, IL: Human Kinetics.

Ryan, M. 2002. *Sports nutrition for endurance athletes.* Boulder, CO: Velo Press.

Sawka, M.N., L.M. Burke, E.R. Eichner, R.J. Maughan, S.J. Montain, and N.S. Stachenfeld. 2007. American College of Sports Medicine position stand. Exercise and fluid replacement. *Medicine and Science in Sports and Exercise* 39(2): 377-390.

Seebohar, B. 2004. *Nutrition periodization for endurance athletes: Taking sports nutrition to the next level.* Boulder, CO: Bull Publishing.

Chapter 5

Dallam, G., and S. Jonas. 2008. *Championship triathlon training.* Champaign, IL: Human Kinetics.

Daniels, J. 2005. *Daniels' running formula: Proven programs 800m to the marathon.* Champaign, IL: Human Kinetics.

Gore, C. (Ed.) 2000. *Physiological tests for elite athletes.* Champaign, IL: Human Kinetics.

Jeukendrup, A. (Ed.) 2002. *High-performance cycling: 28 international experts give you an edge in technique, training, equipment, racing.* Champaign, IL: Human Kinetics.

Lamb, D., and R. Murray. (Ed.) 1997. *Perspectives in exercise science and sports medicine, volume 10. Optimizing sport performance.* Carmel, IN: Cooper Publishing Group.

Martin, D.E., and P.N. Coe. 1997. *Better training for distance runners.* 2nd ed. Champaign, IL: Human Kinetics.

Noakes, T. 2003. *Lore of running.* 4th ed. Champaign, IL: Human Kinetics.

Noakes, T. 2006. The limits of endurance performance. *Basic Research in Cardiology* 101: 408-417.

Sleamaker, R. 1989. *Serious training for serious athletes.* Champaign, IL: Leisure Press.

Chapter 6

Earle, R.W., and T.R. Baechle. 2008. Resistance training and spotting techniques. In R.W. Earle and T.R. Baechle (Eds.), *Essentials of strength training and conditioning.* 3rd ed. Champaign, IL: Human Kinetics.

NSCA. 2008. *Exercise technique manual.* 2nd ed. Champaign, IL: Human Kinetics.

Chapter 7

Bastiaans, J.J., A.B. Van Diemen, T. Veneberg, and A.E. Jeukendrup. 2001. The effects of replacing a portion of endurance training by explosive strength training on performance in trained cyclists. *Eur J Appl Physiol* 86: 79-84.

Bompa, T.O., and G.G. Haff. 2009. *Periodization: Theory and methodology of training.* 5th ed. Champaign, IL: Human Kinetics.

Cressey, E.M., C.A. West, D.P. Tiberio, W.J. Kraemer, and C.M. Maresh. 2007. The effects of ten weeks of lower-body unstable surface training on markers of athletic performance. *J Strength Cond Res* 21: 561-567.

Harre, D. 1982. *Trainingslehre.* Berlin, Germany: Sportverlag.

Issurin, V. 2008. Block periodization versus traditional training theory: A review. *J Sports Med Phys Fitness* 48: 65-75.

Issurin, V. 2008. *Block periodization: Breakthrough in sports training.* In M. Yessis (Ed.), MI: Ultimate Athlete Concepts.

Jackson, N.P., M.S. Hickey, and R.F. Reiser, 2nd. 2007. High resistance/low repetition vs. low resistance/high repetition training: Effects on performance of trained cyclists. *J Strength Cond Res* 21: 289-295.

Jeffreys, I. 2008. Quadrennial planning for the high school athlete. *Strength and Cond J* 30: 74-83.

Jung, A.P. 2003. The impact of resistance training on distance running performance. *Sports Med* 33: 539-552.

Kelly, C.M., A.F. Burnett, and M.J. Newton. 2008. The effect of strength training on three-kilometer performance in recreational women endurance runners. *J Strength Cond Res* 22: 396-403.

Kurz, T. 2001. *Science of sports training.* 2nd ed. Island Pond, VT: Stadion Publishing Company, Inc.

McBride, J.M., P. Cormie, and R. Deane. 2006. Isometric squat force output and muscle activity in stable and unstable conditions. *J Strength Cond Res* 20: 915-918.

Mikkola, J., H. Rusko, A. Nummela, T. Pollari, and K. Hakkinen. 2007. Concurrent endurance and explosive type strength training improves neuromuscular and anaerobic characteristics in young distance runners. *Int J Sports Med* 28: 602-611.

Paavolainen, L., K. Hakkinen, I. Hamalainen, A. Nummela, and H. Rusko. 1999. Explosive-strength training improves 5-km running time by improving running economy and muscle power. *J Appl Physiol* 86: 1527-1533.

Plisk, S.S., and M.H. Stone. 2003. Periodization strategies. *Strength and Cond* 25: 19-37.

Reuter, B.H., and P.S. Hagerman. 2008. Aerobic endurance exercise training. In T.R. Baechle and R.W. Earle (Eds.), *Essentials of strength training and conditioning*. Champaign, IL: Human Kinetics.

Siff, M.C. 2003. *Supertraining*. 6th ed. Denver, CO: Supertraining Institute.

Stanton, R., P.R. Reaburn, and B. Humphries. 2004. The effect of short-term Swiss ball training on core stability and running economy. *J Strength Cond Res* 18: 522-528.

Stone, M.H., M.E. Stone, and W.A. Sands. 2007. *Principles and practice of resistance training*. Champaign, IL: Human Kinetics.

Tanaka, H., and T. Swensen. 1998. Impact of resistance training on endurance performance: A new form of cross-training? *Sports Med* 25: 191-200.

Yamamoto, L.M., R.M. Lopez, J.F. Klau, D.J. Casa, W.J. Kraemer, and C.M. Maresh. 2008. The effects of resistance training on endurance distance running performance among highly trained runners: A systematic review. *J Strength Cond Res* 22: 2036-2044.

Chapter 8

Boyle, M. 2004. *Functional training for sports*. Champaign, IL: Human Kinetics.

Daniels, J. 2005. *Daniels' running formula*. 2nd ed. Champaign, IL: Human Kinetics.

Dolezal, B.A., and J.A. Potteiger. 1996. Resistance training for endurance runners during the off-season. *Strength and Conditioning Journal* 18(3): 7-10.

Foran, B. (Ed.) 2001. *High performance sports conditioning*. Champaign, IL: Human Kinetics.

Friel, J. 2004. *The triathlete's training bible*. 2nd ed. Boulder, CO: VeloPress.

Radcliffe, J.C., and R.C. Farentinos. 1999. *High-powered plyometrics*. Champaign, IL: Human Kinetics.

Romanov, N., and J. Robson. 2004. *Dr. Nicholas Romanov's pose method of running*. Clark Cables, FL: Pose Tech Corp.

Turner, A.M., M. Owings, and J.A. Schwane. 2003. Improvement in running economy after 6 weeks of plyometrics training. *The Journal of Strength and Conditioning Research* 17(1): 60-67.

Whaley, M.H. (Ed.) 2006. *ACSM's guidelines for exercise testing and prescription*. 7th ed. Baltimore, MD; Philadelphia, PA: Lippincott Williams and Wilkins.

Chapter 9

Allen, H., and A. Coggan. 2006. *Training and racing with a power meter.* Boulder, CO: VeloPress.

Borg, G. 1998. *Borg's perceived exertion and pain scales.* Champaign, IL: Human Kinetics.

Browning, R., and R. Sleamaker. 1996. *Serious training for endurance athletes.* 2nd ed. Champaign, IL: Human Kinetics.

Burke, E. 2002. *High tech cycling.* 2nd ed. Champaign, IL: Human Kinetics.

Burke, E. 2002. *Serious cycling.* 2nd ed. Champaign, IL: Human Kinetics.

Friel, J. 2003. *The cyclist's training bible.* 3rd ed. Boulder, CO: VeloPress.

Pruitt, A., and F. Matheny. 2006. *Andy Pruitt's complete medical guide for cyclists.* Boulder, CO: VeloPress.

Trombley, A. 2005. *Serious mountain biking.* Champaign, IL: Human Kinetics.

Wenzel, K., and R. Wenzel. 2003. *Bike racing 101.* Champaign, IL: Human Kinetics.

Zinn, L. 2004. *Zinn's cycling primer.* Boulder, CO: VeloPress.

Chapter 10

Dallam, G., and S. Jonas. 2008. *Championship triathlon training.* Champaign, IL: Human Kinetics.

Hannula, D. 2003. *Coaching swimming successfully.* 2nd ed. Champaign, IL: Human Kinetics.

Laughlin, T. 1996. *Total immersion: The revolutionary way to swim better, faster, easier.* New York: Fireside.

Maglischo, E. 2003. *Swimming fastest: The essential reference on technique, training and program design.* Champaign, IL: Human Kinetics.

Chapter 11

Bompa, T. 1999. *Periodization theory and methodology of training.* Champaign, IL: Human Kinetics.

Bompa, T., and M. Carrera. 2005. *Periodization training for sports.* Champaign, IL: Human Kinetics.

Colwin, C. 2002. *Breakthrough swimming.* Champaign, IL: Human Kinetics.

Dallam, G., and S. Jonas. 2008. *Championship triathlon training.* Champaign, IL: Human Kinetics.

Evans, M. 2003. *Triathlete's edge.* Champaign, IL: Human Kinetics.

Friel, J. 2008. *Triathlete's training bible.* Boulder, CO: Velo Press.

Gambetta, V. 2007. *Athletic development: The art and science of functional sports conditioning.* Champaign, IL: Human Kinetics.

Maglischo, E. 2003. *Swimming fastest.* Champaign, IL: Human Kinetics.

Prehn, T. 2004. *Racing tactics for cyclists.* Boulder, CO: Velo Press.

Index

Note: The italicized *f* and *t* following page numbers refer to figures and tables, respectively.

About the NSCA

The **National Strength and Conditioning Association (NSCA)** is the world's leading organization in the field of sport conditioning. Drawing on the resources and expertise of more than 30,000 professionals in strength training and conditioning, sport science, performance research, education, and sports medicine, the NSCA is the world's most trusted source of knowledge and training guidelines for coaches and athletes. The NSCA provides the crucial link between the lab and the field.

About the Editor

Ben Reuter, PhD, CSCS*D, ATC, is an associate professor in the department of exercise science and sport studies at California University of Pennsylvania. Ben earned his doctorate in exercise physiology from Auburn University, and he earned his masters, with an emphasis in athletic training, from Old Dominion University. Ben is also a certified strength and conditioning specialist, with distinction, and holds a certification from the Pilates Method Alliance. Ben is an associate editor for the *Strength and Conditioning Journal*, a journal of the NSCA. His research interests include injury prevention and performance enhancement for age-group endurance athletes. Ben has presented for a number 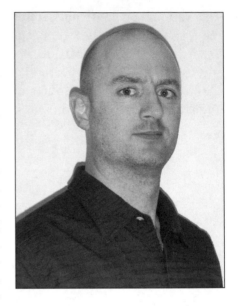 of professional organizations regionally, nationally, and internationally, including a trip to China to present for the NSCA in the summer of 2009.

About the Contributors

Stephanie Burgess, BS, is a graduate of West Virginia University. She was an undergraduate research intern in the division of exercise physiology at the West Virginia University School of Medicine at Morgantown. She was a member of the West Virginia University women's soccer team from 2004 to 2008.

Denny DePriest, RSCC, has facilitated physical education and health classes for the last three and a half years at Kaiserslautern High School in Kaiserslautern, Germany, for the U.S. Department of Defense. He is the former coach of the USA Triathlon resident and U23 national select team. He has presented at the NSCA European conference and maintains the following certifications: certified strength and conditioning specialist (from NSCA), level 3 elite triathlon coach (from USA Triathlon), level 2 expert cycling coach (from USA Cycling), and level 2 expert track and field coach (from USA Track and Field).

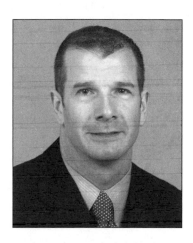

Jason Gootman, MS, CSCS, co-director of Tri-Hard, coaches triathletes and other endurance athletes in the Boston area, throughout New England, and around the world. Tri-Hard athletes include in their ranks several professional triathletes as well as numerous qualifiers for the Age-Group World and National Championships (including a world and national champion), the Ironman 70.3 World Championship, and the Ironman World Championship. Jason has a master's degree in exercise physiology, and he is a certified triathlon coach (USA Triathlon) and a certified strength and conditioning specialist (NSCA).

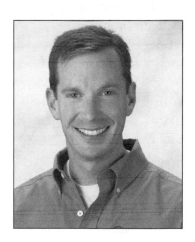

Greg Haff, PhD, CSCS*D, FNSCA, is a senior lecturer and course coordinator for the masters of strength and conditioning program at Edith Cowan University at Joondalup, Western Australia. A level 3 cycling coach, he has served as a strength and conditioning consultant for several collegiate cyclists, track athletes, and soccer athletes. In 2001, the NSCA recognized him as the Young Investigator of the Year for his work in sport science.

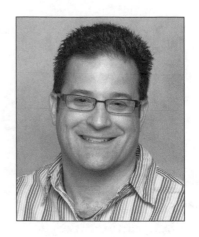

Neal Henderson, MS, CSCS, is the director of sport science at the Boulder Center for Sports Medicine in Boulder, Colorado. Neal earned his bachelor's degree in exercise and sport science from Penn State University and earned his master's degree in kinesiology at the University of Colorado at Boulder. He is an elite level certified coach by both USA Cycling and USA Triathlon and has coached multiple world champions in triathlon and cycling (from juniors to masters and from U23 to elite). He is a retired professional triathlete himself and an amateur and masters national and world championship medalist in track cycling and XTERRA triathlon, respectively.

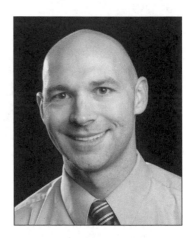

Will Kirousis, CSCS, co-director of Tri-Hard, coaches triathletes and other endurance athletes in the Boston area, throughout New England, and around the world. Tri-Hard athletes include in their ranks several professional triathletes as well as numerous qualifiers for the Age-Group World and National Championships (including a world and national champion), the Ironman 70.3 World Championship, and the Ironman World Championship. Will has a bachelor's degree in exercise science and is a USA Triathlon certified coach, USA Cycling certified coach, and NSCA certified strength and conditioning specialist.

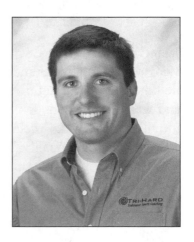

Peter Melanson, MS, CSCS*D, RSCC*D, is currently the education department manager for the National Strength and Conditioning Association (NSCA). He recently returned to the NSCA after a three-year term as the head strength and conditioning coach for the U.S. Olympic Committee (USOC) based in Colorado Springs, where he oversaw all three USOC training center S&C facilities. Before his work at the USOC, he was the educational programs coordinator for the NSCA. His experience includes six years as the assistant strength and conditioning coach for the U.S. Air Force Academy. He has trained elite collegiate, amateur, and professional athletes, including athletes for the New York Jets (NFL) and the University of Tennessee Volunteers. Mr. Melanson also served as the national director of strength/conditioning and advanced rehab for HealthSouth, while developing and operating their Human Performance Center.

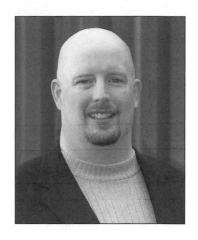

Bob Seebohar, MS, RD, CSSD, CSCS, is a nationally known (and board certified) specialist in sport dietetics, a certified strength and conditioning specialist through NSCA, and a USA Triathlon certified elite coach. He was previously the director of sport nutrition at the University of Florida and, most recently, a sport dietitian for the U.S. Olympic Committee. In 2008, Bob traveled to the Summer Olympics with Team USA and was the sport dietitian for the Olympic triathlon team. He currently owns his own businesses: Fuel-4mance, a sport nutrition consulting company, and Elite Multisport Coaching, which provides endurance coaching services to athletes of all ages and abilities. Bob has an undergraduate degree in exercise and sport science, a master's degree in health and exercise science, and a second master's degree in food science and human nutrition.

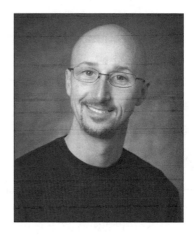

Suzie Snyder, MS, CSCS, is a triathlon coach and tactical human performance coach. Suzie earned her bachelor's degree in physical education and a master's degree in exercise science (with a concentration in strength and conditioning) from Springfield College. Suzie is an NSCA certified strength and conditioning specialist, USA Triathlon level 1 coach, and USA Cycling level 3 coach. She has experience as a collegiate athlete in cross country and track and field. Additionally, she spent two years as a Division III collegiate assistant coach in women's track and field. Suzie is now in her second year as a professional triathlete; she has competed and earned honors in XTERRA and ITU National and World Championships.

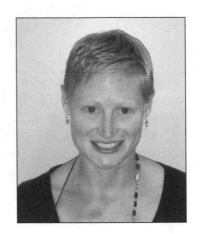

Randy Wilber, PhD, FACSM, works with U.S. Olympic team athletes from a variety of sports and advises them on the scientific and practical aspects of training. He has provided support for Team USA athletes at six Olympic Games and two Pan American Games. Dr. Wilber's research interests include evaluating the effects of environmental factors on elite athletic performance. He has authored the book *Altitude Training and Athletic Performance: Theory and Practice* and coedited *Exercise-Induced Asthma: Pathophysiology and Treatment* (2002).

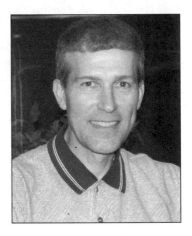

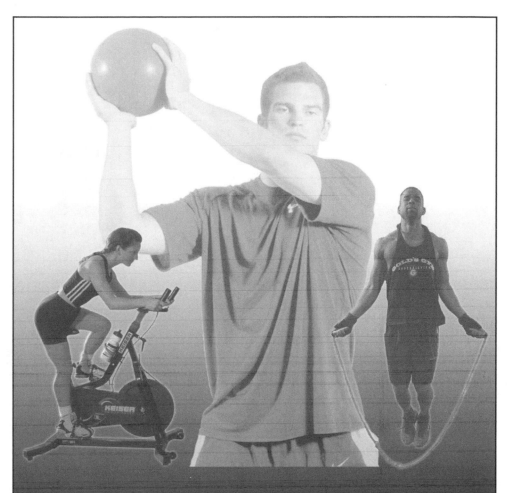